TRANSFORM YOUR BODY WITH WEIGHTS

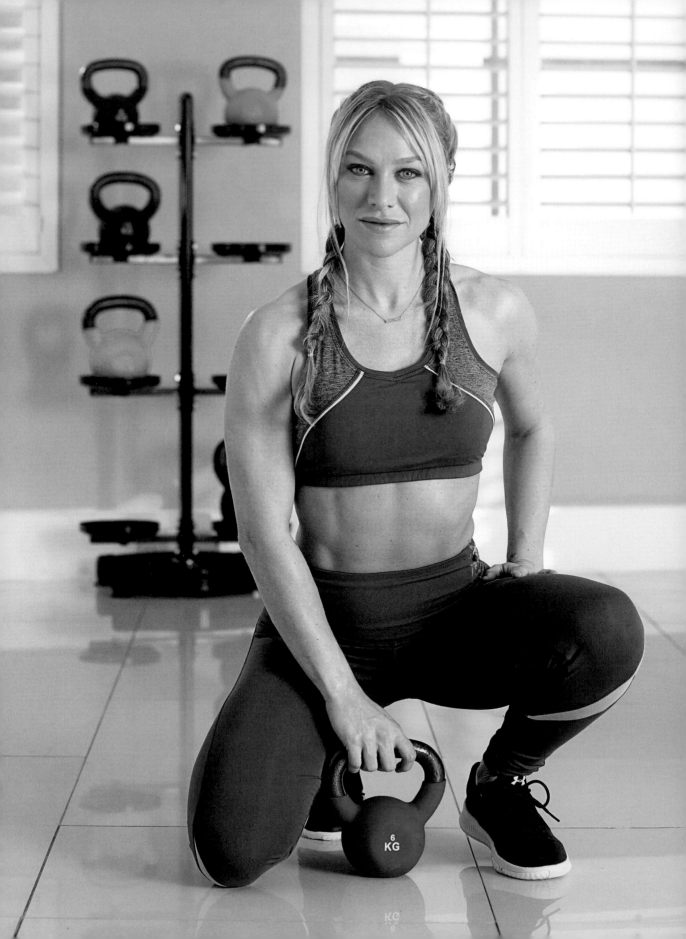

TRANSFORM YOUR BODY WITH WEIGHTS
CHLOE MADELEY

Complete workout and meal plans,
from beginner to advanced

BANTAM PRESS

LONDON · NEW YORK · TORONTO · SYDNEY · AUCKLAND

TRANSWORLD PUBLISHERS
61–63 Uxbridge Road, London W5 5SA
www.penguin.co.uk

Transworld is part of the Penguin Random House group
of companies whose addresses can be found at global.
penguinrandomhouse.com

Penguin
Random House
UK

First published in Great Britain in 2019 by Bantam Press
an imprint of Transworld Publishers

Project editor: Jo Roberts-Miller
Design: Smith & Gilmour
Cover and exercise photography: Sam Riley
Food photography: Smith & Gilmour
Food styling: Lisa Harrison & Anna Burges-Lumsden

Every effort has been made to obtain the necessary permissions
with reference to copyright material, both illustrative and quoted.
We apologize for any omissions in this respect and will be pleased
to make the appropriate acknowledgements in any future edition.

A CIP catalogue record for this book is available from the
British Library.

ISBN 9781787631601

Typeset in Museo Slab 9.75/14pt by Smith & Gilmour
Printed and bound in China by C&C Offset Printing Co., Ltd

Penguin Random House is committed to a sustainable future for
our business, our readers and our planet. This book is made from
Forest Stewardship Council® certified paper.

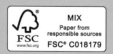

FSC
www.fsc.org
MIX
Paper from
responsible sources
FSC® C018179

1 3 5 7 9 10 8 6 4 2

CONTENTS

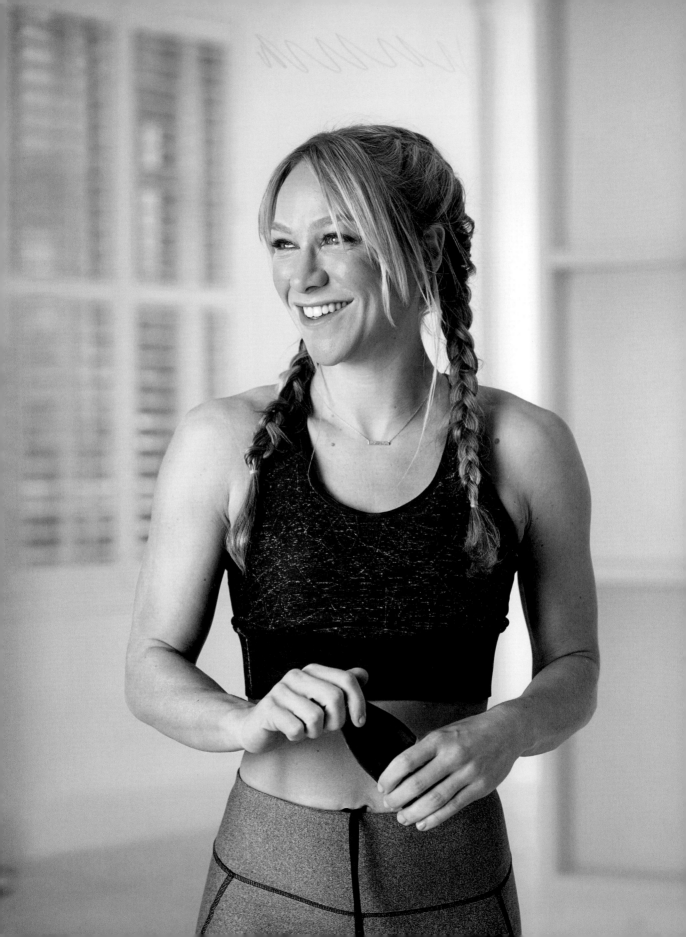

INTRODUCTION

Seven years ago, I truly believed that I *hated* exercise.

I bunked every P.E. and Games lesson in school, I would go for a run *only* if I was feeling stressed or anxious, and not once did I find myself enjoying exercise.

When I started dating a Personal Trainer, there wasn't a valid excuse *not* to go to the gym with him, so off I trudged, planning how to impress him while simultaneously doing as little work as humanly possible.

For our very first training session, he took me over to the Smith Machine and taught me how to squat. It sounds too good to be true but, within minutes, I was hooked.

I had never done exercise like this before – exercise that actually felt good *while* you were doing it. Exercise that I *wanted* to do for a full hour, and do again the next day.

Looking back, I can honestly say that weight lifting has *completely* changed my life. Now, I enjoy exercise, I've increased my fitness and have become physically strong, feeling accomplished, feeling challenged, seeing aesthetic definition… from the inside out, my entire life has been greatly enhanced by this one, specific discipline.

And with every passing year, I watch the stigma around female weight lifting melt away. The weights section of my gym has gradually climbed from being 10% female to 50% female. Women now understand that lifting weights doesn't make them 'bulky', it makes them 'toned', and the idea that the weights section of the gym is 'the men's area' is now firmly a thing of the past.

However, there are still a lot of women out there who *want* to lift weights, but are too intimidated to try. A lot of these women may be *intrigued* by the results of this type of training, but are too fearful of becoming 'bulky' to get off the treadmill. So, yes, there is still an element of truth in the idea that females fear weight lifting, BUT it has now become the exception, not the rule.

Now men *and* women are aware of the physical *and* mental benefits of weight lifting and are becoming advocates of the sport. These benefits include:

» Weight management

» Increased muscle mass

» Aesthetic body transformation through altered body composition (fat loss coupled with increased muscle mass, aka 'toning')

» Basal metabolic rate increase (up to 10%)

» Increased bone density (aiding anti-aging and preventing osteoporosis)

» Anti-aging physicality (bettered movement control, physical function, physical performance and speed)

» Improvement in cardiovascular health

» Reduced blood pressure

» Management of chronic pain

» Studied and now proven improvements in overall mood, anxiety and depressive tendencies

These are just some of the reasons why I lift weights, but the main reason? It's *fun.* While I do enjoy cardio, long winter walks, sweaty circuit training and swimming, absolutely nothing gets me as excited as weight lifting – it's challenging, it's exciting and it's *rewarding.*

So, here we are... welcome to *Transform Your Body with Weights* – a weight-lifting guide for every level of lifter – even those of you who've never lifted a weight in your life!

HOW TO USE THIS BOOK

There are four main sections to this book.

>> In the first, **The Weight-training Plans**, you choose your lifting level – Beginner, Intermediate or Advanced – then your lifting goal – Endurance (great for cardio bunnies), Hypertrophy (great for muscle building) or Strength (great for strength and performance).

>> In the second, **Your Physique Goal**, you can choose a diet and cardio plan to achieve a physique goal, such as fat loss or muscle building. However, you can leave this section out and simply use the book as a weight-lifting guide.

>> In the third, **The Food Bible and Recipes**, you marry your food intake to your training and / or physique goal. All the recipes have calorie and macro breakdowns so, if you track, you can manipulate the ingredients and quantities when and where necessary.

PLEASE NOTE:

ALL MY RECIPES SERVE ONE

>> Finally, in the last section, **Recovery**, I explain how best to let your body recover when following a weight-lifting plan, in order to get the best internal *and* external results.

UNDERSTANDING FORM BEFORE YOU BEGIN

Form is your physical ability to perform a lift correctly. For example, a squat requires a straight back at all times, bending *only* at the hips and knees. Your knees should be pointing forwards, directly above your toes at all times, and when you have reached your full range of motion (as low as you can go), you stand up straight again, pushing down through your heels. If you were to bend forwards, or allow your knees to invert, or if you were to push up through your toes, all of these would indicate bad form.

Once your form is near perfect, *then* you can focus on adding weight and / or changing your sets and reps ranges (see pages 14–15). This is often referred to as 'overload' and is pivotal to progressing your muscle growth and / or strength and performance goals.

No matter what your goal (endurance, hypertrophy or strength), form should *always* be primary, weight secondary.

CHOOSING YOUR
WEIGHT-TRAINING GOAL

» Endurance Training
(the muscle's ability to generate force repeatedly)

Endurance training is perfect for those wanting to increase their 'functional' training abilities, such as triathletes, distance runners and rowers. If you are a cardio bunny looking to implement some weight lifting to assist your sport, then endurance is perfect for you.

Endurance training is typically 2–3 sets of 15+ reps before muscle exhaust. (*Reps are how many times you perform the exercise. For example: 15 squats = 15 reps. Sets are how many times you repeat the reps. For example: 3 sets = 15 reps performed 3 times, with a short rest between sets.*)

» Hypertrophy Training
(the growth of a muscle)

Hypertrophy training (muscle building) is for those wanting to increase muscle mass and is my favourite form of weight lifting. If you have a physique goal and are looking for aesthetic muscular results, hypertrophy is for you.

Hypertrophy is typically 3–4 sets of 6–12 reps before muscle exhaust.

» Strength Training
(the muscle's ability to generate force against resistance)

Strength training (or Powerlifting) is perfect for those wanting to increase their physical strength and really enjoy their weight lifting. It traditionally only calls for 3 exercises: squat, deadlift and bench press, as these are the competition lifts. However, in recent years, 2 common exercises have been added to the training – the military press and the barbell row.

Hypertrophy 'accessory work' (see below) has also become a common theme in strength training, so if you'd like to include some hypertrophy in your strength routine, that is perfectly acceptable.

Strength training is typically 1–5 sets of between 1–5 reps, before muscle exhaust (meaning you lift very heavy weights and have 1–5 reps MAX before you exhaust).

It is worth pointing out that even though you should be focusing on one particular goal – endurance, hypertrophy or strength – *each* discipline can help the other. For example, **endurance** can greatly impact and improve both **hypertrophy** and **strength**, especially when it comes to those big compound lifts, such as squats, which require overall physical fitness. **Hypertrophy** training can greatly improve your **strength** goals, as the more muscle you have, the stronger you are in your lift. **Strength** can improve your **hypertrophy**, as the stronger you are, the more weight you can shift in your sets and reps range. And around and around we go!

As a result, although I recommend you choose one goal and stick to it *most* of the time, if you fancy throwing in the odd curveball exercise, session, or even week of training, it can greatly enhance your overall results. This is often referred to as **Accessory Work**. On the other hand, in strength training, if you take a week away from overload and allow your body to recover, this is called a **Deload Week**.

LIFTING RULES TO LIVE BY

Whatever goal you choose, you will be lifting weights
and there are some important lifting rules to live by...

>> Gym instructors and Personal Trainers are paid to show you how to use the equipment in the gym properly – use them if you need to.

>> YouTube is a good source of visual references for lifts and how to perform them correctly.

>> Ask friends or family who know how to lift if you can shadow them at the gym to learn the right techniques.

>> Watch people on the machines to get an idea of how they work and how to use them before you jump on.

>> *Never* be intimidated by the weights section in a gym; everyone in there was a beginner at some point, and even the pros are still learning!

>> Remember to stretch before and after every session (see pages 17–27); this will improve your range of motion and recovery.

>> Your body can only do what it can do, never force your range of motion beyond what it is capable of doing.

>> Remember that technique is more important than weight when it comes to lifting – focus on perfecting your form *before* you increase your weight.

>> Make sure to breathe during your set – deep breaths in when relaxing the muscle, long breaths out when forcing the muscle.

>> Start with a light weight and only increase when you feel you can.

>> As soon as you feel you can increase the weight, be brave and do so.

>> Never lock out *any* joint when lifting, always keep a *slight bend* in your joints.

>> Mind to muscle connection is very real – *think* of the muscle that is meant to be working during the exercise.

》 If you cannot feel the exercise working the right muscle, play around with positions and contractions until you have a better idea of how to make it best work for you. Alternatively, warm up the intended muscle by contracting it several times *before* you lift. For example, I always do an unweighted glute bridge hold before I train my lower body, as I am quad dominant and I need to wake my glutes up.

》 Bad form is dangerous – if you know you are doing something wrong, stop immediately and ask for help. However, if you need to change your stance in order to feel the right muscle working (for example, widening your stance in a lift), and **you know there is no physical danger in doing so**, then go for it.

》 Feel free to play around with weights, sets and reps. Yes, I have detailed a very specific plan for you, but if you want to try something new for a session (or take a week off your plan to try something different), it will only help your overall learning, training and results – so go for it!

》 No matter what your goal (**endurance**, **hypertrophy** or **strength**), 'overload' is key to progress – this means increasing weight, sets and / or reps over time. Adding difficulty is *pivotal* to progression.

》 Finally, rest is just as important as training when it comes to internal *and* external results. Listen to your body and implement rest days as and when you need them. (See Part 4 for more on recovery – see pages 245–249.)

SETS, REPS AND REST GUIDE

In this book I recommend a variety of sets, reps and rest ranges depending on your:

>> Lifting level
(Beginner / Intermediate / Advanced)

>> Chosen goal
(Endurance / Hypertrophy / Strength)

>> Stage of training
(Week 1, 2, 3 or 4)

The different levels, goals and stages require different sets, reps and rest ranges for different reasons.

I want you to understand *why* you're doing what you're doing so I'm going to explain how these ranges work...

Basic Sets, Reps and Rest

Your basic sets, reps and rest range will depend on your chosen goal:

>> **Endurance** – 2–3 sets of 15+ reps with *as little rest* between sets as possible

>> **Hypertrophy** – 3–4 sets of 6–12 reps with 1–2 minutes rest between sets

>> **Strength** – 1–5 sets of 1–5 reps with as much rest between sets as needed

Set to Exhaust
(Isometric Hold)

You will see the instruction '1 set to exhaust' with exercises such as the plank (see page 103) – this is also called an Isometric Hold. There are 3 ways in which muscles are worked:

>> Concentric (shortening of the muscle, such as the lifting of the weight in a bicep curl – see page 47)

>> Eccentric (lengthening of the muscle, such as the lowering of the weight in a bicep curl – see page 47)

>> Isometric (contraction of the muscle without any movement, such as the plank – see page 103)

Isometric Holds cannot be done with every exercise, but when performed appropriately they can be a *great* way to fully exhaust the muscle with one simple set, as well as improving your overall physical strength and endurance.

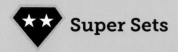 ## Super Sets

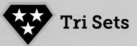 ## Tri Sets

Super sets are simply 2 exercises (such as a shoulder press and a push-up) performed to their instructed reps back-to-back (without any rest between the 2 exercises). Having performed both exercises, you then rest before the next set, and continue for however many sets are instructed.

For example, for a super set of 3 sets of 12 reps of shoulder presses and lateral raises, you should do 12 reps of a shoulder press followed *immediately* by 12 reps of a lateral raise, before resting for 1–2 minutes in preparation for the next set.

Super sets can be done in the Endurance and Hypertrophy ranges, but Strength training requires a lot more energy *and* rest, so strength exercises should always be performed as basic sets and reps.

Super sets are a great way to save time, exhaust the muscle and, if performed using agonist / antagonist muscles (biceps and triceps, for example), can provide extremely effective training sessions.

Tri sets are simply 3 exercises (such as wide grip pull-ups, close grip pull-ups and tricep dips) performed to their instructed reps back-to-back (without any rest between the exercises). Having performed all 3 exercises, you then rest before the next set and continue for however many sets are instructed.

For example, with a tri set of 3 sets of 12 reps of shoulder presses, lateral raises and front raises, you should do 12 reps of a shoulder press, followed *immediately* by 12 reps of a lateral raise, followed *immediately* by 12 reps of a front raise, before resting for 1–2 minutes in preparation for the next set.

Tri sets can be done in the Endurance and Hypertrophy ranges but Strength training requires a lot more energy *and* rest, so should be performed as basic sets and reps.

Tri sets are a great way to save time, exhaust the muscle, and can provide extremely effective training sessions.

There are other sets, reps and rest ranges (Forced Reps and Negative Reps, for example, that can greatly aid Strength training), but the fact is that *most* of us don't need to *over*-complicate or *over*-experiment with our training routines. While the Endurance, Hypertrophy and Strength plans can be played around with in order to benefit one another, you can absolutely go too far and hinder both your training and your intended results in the process. Remember that when it comes to making progress, the main factor in any training plan is *overload* (added sets, reps, and / or weight). You will not progress if you do not change or increase *something* en route – after a while, the body *really does* adapt.

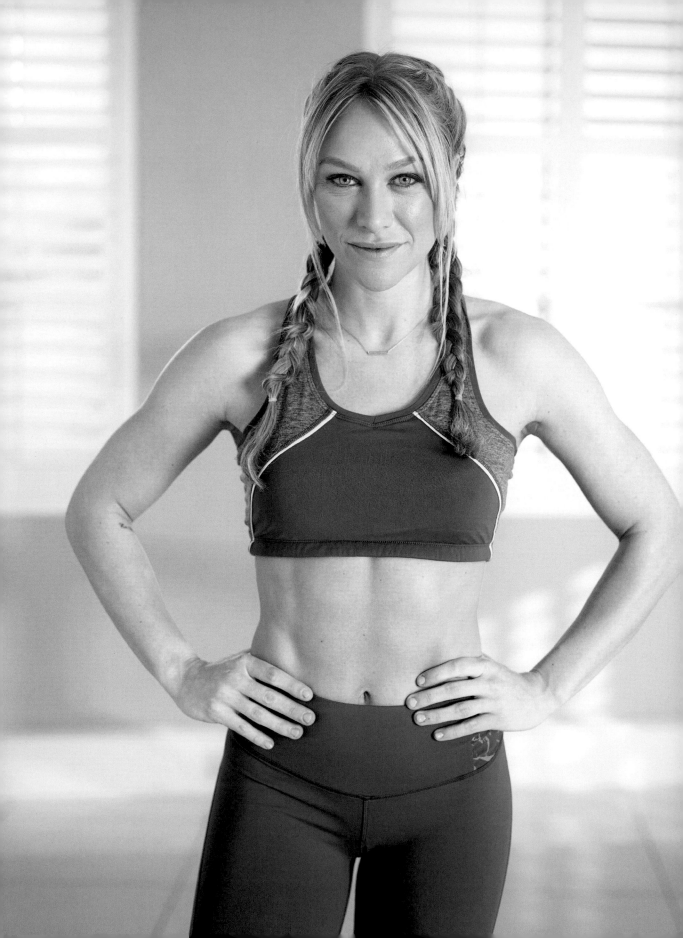

STRETCHING

You *must* warm up before and cool down after every training session.

Think of your body as a piece of chewing gum – if it's cold and you bend it, it will snap. If it's warm and you bend it, it will be supple and move.

Please note:
Warm-up stretches are performed dynamically, meaning with a slow and gentle bouncy movement.

To make a stretch dynamic, hold the position and perform a gentle bounce as you do so, for 8–10 repetitions.

Cool-down stretches are performed statically, meaning still.

To make a stretch static, hold the position still for 8–10 seconds.

Some of the stretches are for warming up only, most are for both warming up and cooling down. All the stretches are labelled so you know which are which.

SHOULDER STRETCH

WARM UP ONLY Stand up straight with your feet hip-width apart. Let your arms hang down by your sides. Place one hand across your body, resting it gently on the opposite side of your chest. Lift your other arm out in front of you, then slowly raise it vertically up into the air. Let it gently continue a circle behind your body, and complete the circle by letting it a hang by your side where it started. Repeat this circular motion 8–10 times, then perform with the opposite arm.

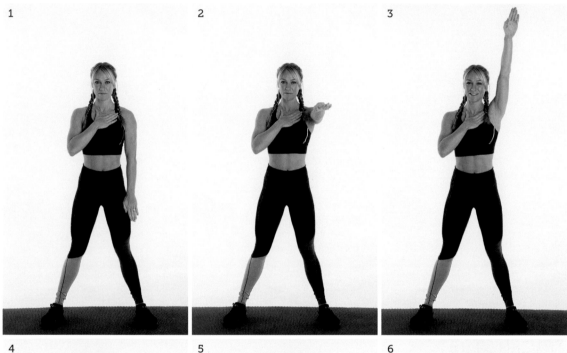

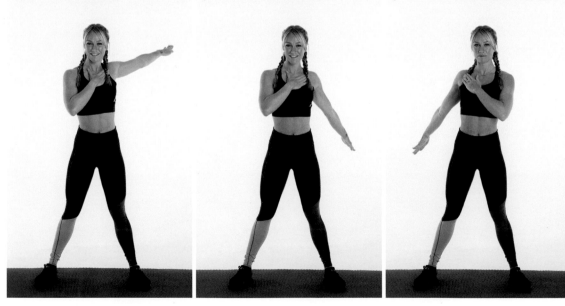

SHOULDER STRETCH

WARM UP & COOL DOWN

Stand up straight with your feet hip-width apart. Let your arms hang down by your sides. Lift one arm out in front of you. Reach your opposite hand across your body, under your elbow, and flatten your hand behind the extended arm's shoulder. Slowly and gently use your flattened hand to push against the back of the elbow, extending the arm across your upper body, so it is horizontal across your chest. Repeat with the opposite arm.

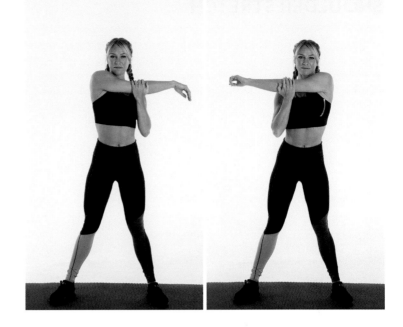

TRICEP STRETCH

WARM UP & COOL DOWN

Stand up straight with your feet hip-width apart. Lift one arm up into the air and then allow your forearm to hang down gently behind your head and neck. Using your opposite hand, gently grasp the back of your elbow / tricep area. Slowly push against this area so you feel a pull / stretch in your arm. Repeat with the opposite arm.

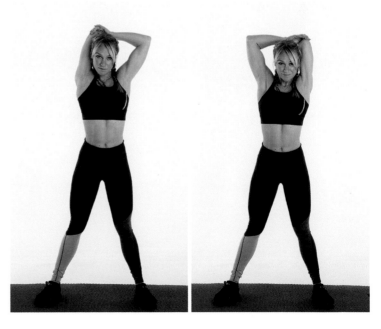

WRIST STRETCH

WARM UP ONLY Stand up straight with your feet hip-width apart. Extend both arms out to the sides (maintain a slight bend in your elbows). Slowly and gently roll your wrists outwards and inwards, in clockwise and anticlockwise movements. Continue this movement for 8–10 seconds.

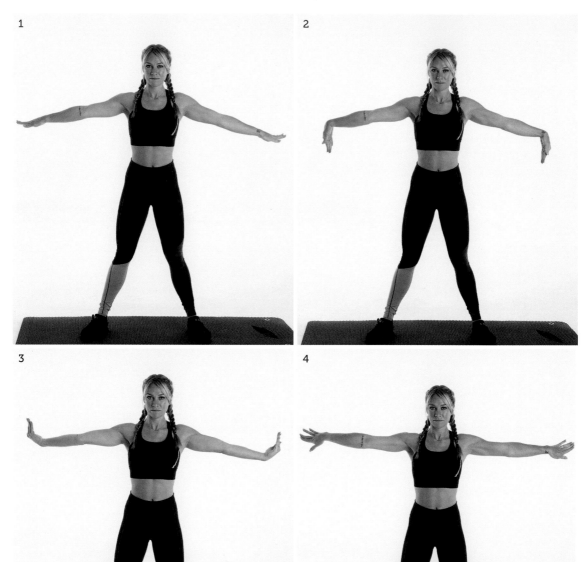

1

2

3

4

NECK STRETCH

WARM UP ONLY Stand up straight with your feet hip-width apart. Look straight ahead, then slowly and gently turn your head to one side, before coming back to centre. Then slowly and gently turn your head to the opposite side, before coming back to centre once again. Then look down, before coming back to centre, and finally look up, before coming back to centre again.

1   2   3

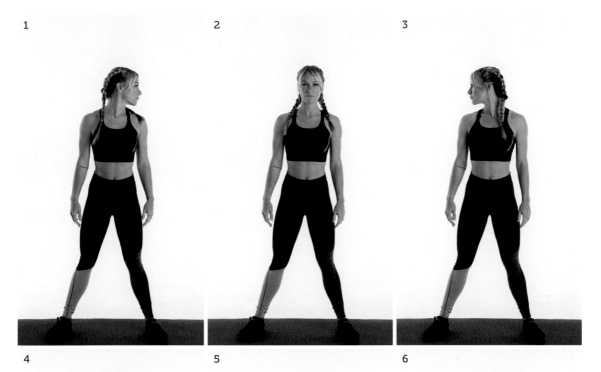

4   5   6

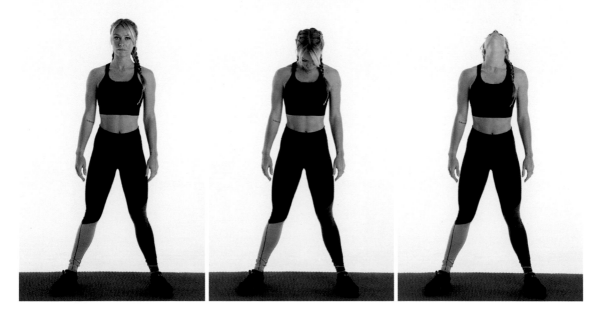

QUAD STRETCH

WARM UP & COOL DOWN
You may need to hold on to something to keep your balance while doing this. Stand up straight with your feet together. Bend one knee, lifting one foot up behind your body, and grasp the foot with your hand. Slowly and gently pull your foot upwards, so you feel a pull/stretch down the front of your leg/quad. Repeat with your opposite leg.

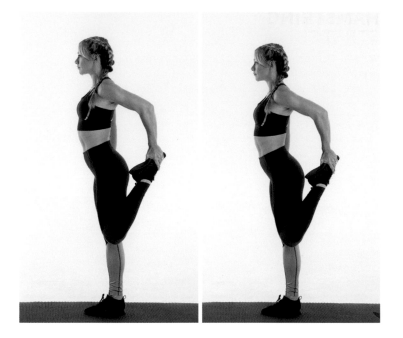

KNEE CIRCLES

WARM UP ONLY Stand with your feet together and bend down slightly so your hands fit in between your knees. Gently circle your knees in a clockwise direction 8 times, before repeating in the opposite direction.

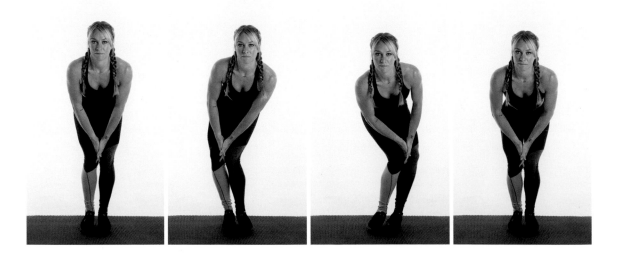

HAMSTRING STRETCH

WARM UP & COOL DOWN
Stand up straight with your feet together. Slowly and gently bend one knee (rest your hands on this knee to balance or, alternatively, place your hands on your hips). Slowly and gently stretch the opposite leg out in front of you, resting on the heel, toes pointing upwards. Keep your shoulders relaxed and feel the stretch in the back of your outstretched leg/hamstring. Repeat this movement with your opposite leg. Repeat with each leg 8–10 times to warm up. Hold each stretch for 8–10 seconds to cool down.

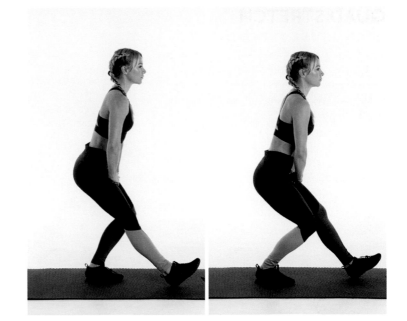

HIP OPENER

WARM UP & COOL DOWN Stand with your legs wide apart, toes facing outwards. Keeping your back straight at all times, slowly and gently come down into a low squat. Rest your elbows on your knees for balance. Slowly and gently lean to the right, stretching out your left hip. Repeat on each side 8–10 times to warm up. Hold each stretch for 8–10 seconds to cool down.

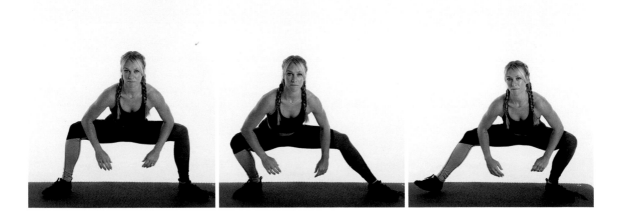

GLUTE STRETCH

WARM UP & COOL DOWN

Stand on your left leg and place your right ankle on top of your left thigh. Lower yourself down into a seated position – you will feel the stretch in the right side of your glute (buttocks). You can help the stretch by pressing gently on top of your right knee. Repeat with the opposite leg. If you have trouble keeping your balance, you can find something to hold on to.

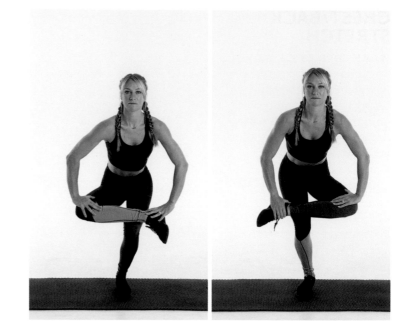

CALF STRETCH

WARM UP & COOL DOWN

Stand up straight with your feet together. Place your hands on your hips and lunge forward on one leg, as far as you can within your natural range. Keeping your back leg straight, try and push your back heel down to the ground – you should feel a stretch/pull in your calf muscle. Repeat with the opposite leg.

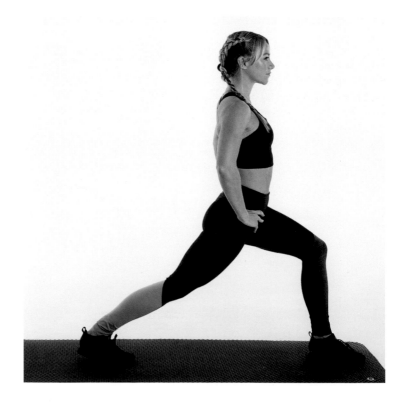

CHEST/BACK STRETCH

WARM UP ONLY Stand up straight with your feet hip-width apart. Raise your arms up to chest height and slowly and gently try to touch your elbows behind your back, within your natural range. Slowly and gently bring your arms back in front of your chest and cross your arms, almost like you are giving yourself a hug. Repeat this movement 8–10 times.

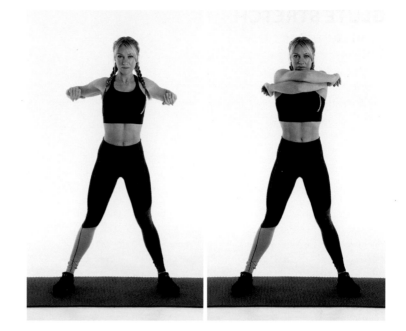

CHEST/BACK STRETCH

WARM UP & COOL DOWN Stand up straight with your feet hip-width apart. Let your arms hang loose at your sides before gently holding your hands behind your back. Slowly and gently extend your arms behind you, within your natural range, and try to pull your shoulders back and push your chest out.

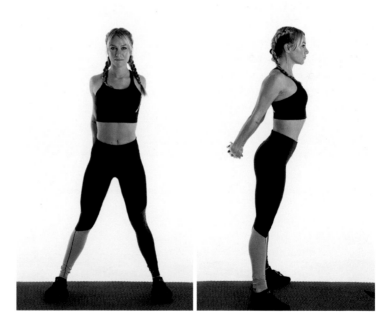

ANKLE ROLLS

WARM UP ONLY Using a simple circular motion, rotate each foot at the ankle for 10 circuits in each direction.

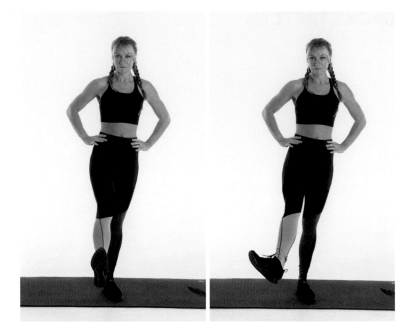

AB STRETCH

WARM UP & COOL DOWN Stand up straight with your feet hip-width apart. Raise your arms up above your head and lace your fingers together, palms facing the ceiling. Extend your upper body upwards as much as you can within your range. You should feel a stretch up the front of your torso and also up the back of your spine. After holding this position for 8–10 seconds, keep your back straight and slowly and gently bend to one side. You will feel a pull along the side of your torso. Repeat on the opposite side.

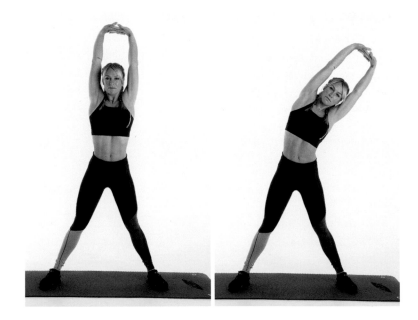

BACK STRETCH

WARM UP & COOL DOWN

Stand up straight with your feet wide apart. Crossing your arms in front of you, let them wrap all the way around your chest, like you are giving yourself a hug. With your hands flat against the backs of your shoulders, perform a gentle pull – you should feel this stretch in the centre of your back. Slowly bend down, creating a convex shape with your spine.

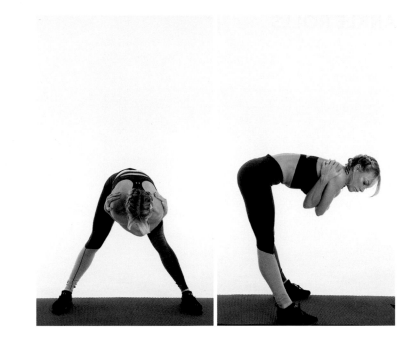

BICEP STRETCH

WARM UP & COOL DOWN

Stand up straight with your feet hip-width apart. Extend one arm out in front of you, your fingertips pointing upwards, your palm facing forwards. Place your opposite arm slightly above the other, your fingertips facing downwards, your palm facing inwards. Slide this hand over the other and slowly and gently pull. You will feel a stretch along the inside of your arm. Repeat with the opposite arm.

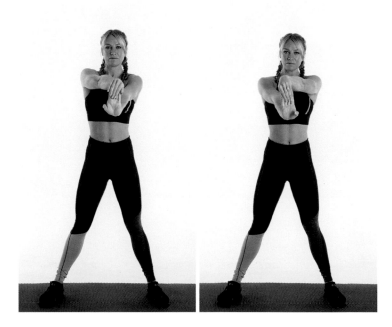

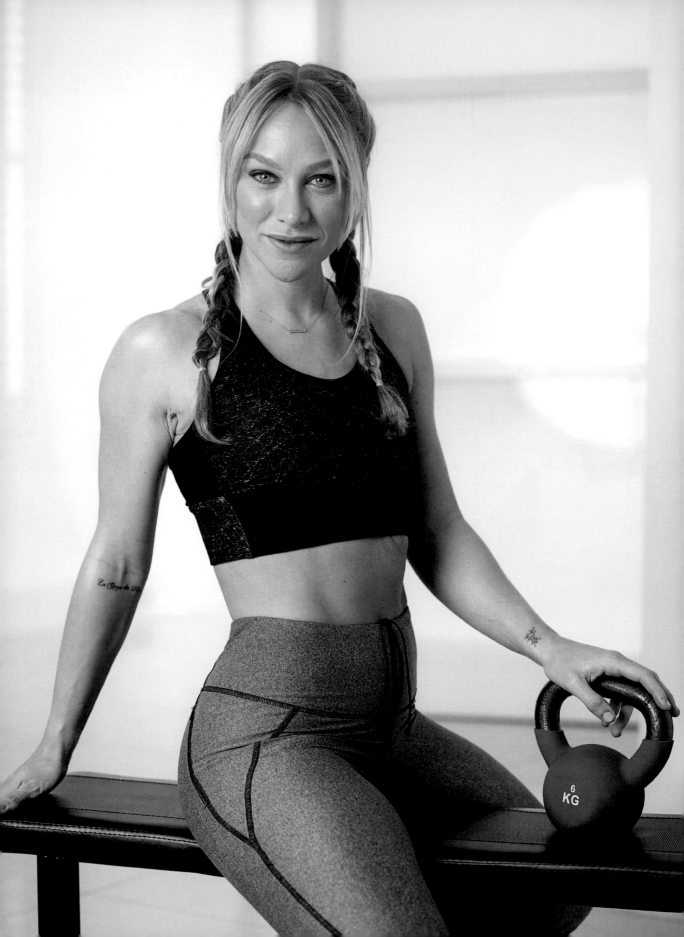

THE WEIGHT-TRAINING PLANS

BEGINNER

First and foremost, let me start by assuring you that you are not required to throw yourself in at the deep end of the weight-lifting pool. In fact, what I want from you beginners is the complete opposite – I want you to use this guide to get your feet wet and focus on form.

One of my favourite expressions in the weight-lifting world is: *'Start as you mean to continue.'* In other words: *'Get your form right now and worry about the weights later.'*

I want you to learn how to execute a movement properly first, without worrying about the weight you are lifting.

Form is the most important factor when it comes to weight lifting. Without good, safe form, you are more than likely going to:

» Hurt yourself
» Expend a lot of energy doing ineffective training
» End up having to unlearn and then relearn appropriate form later

Obviously, something as visual as form is very tricky to teach in a book. You'll find exercise imagery and explanations throughout the plan but other visual aids will go a long way towards helping you understand what these exercises should look like. For example:

» YouTube
» Gym Instructors
» Personal Trainers
» Friends or family who lift
» Even just watching other people in the gym

If you can watch somebody lift *properly*, it will be a lot easier for you to recreate it later.

Only your body can tell you how heavy a weight you should be lifting. Obviously, as a beginner, I urge you to start small. The goal here is to get you used to an exercise with a little additional weight, not get you used to a weight alone. What I mean by this is that:

The exercise is your *primary* concern and the weight is your *secondary* concern.

Once you feel that you have form down, be brave and increase your weight.

Choosing Your Weight-training Goal

» **Endurance Training** *(the muscle's ability to generate force repeatedly)* is perfect for those wanting to increase their 'functional' training abilities, such as triathletes, distance runners and rowers. If you are a cardio bunny looking to implement some weight lifting to assist your sport, then endurance is perfect for you.

» **Hypertrophy Training** *(the growth of a muscle)* is perfect for those wanting to increase visible muscle mass, and is my favourite form of weight lifting. If you are looking for aesthetic muscular results, hypertrophy is for you.

» **Strength Training** *(the muscle's ability to generate force against resistance)* or powerlifting is perfect for those wanting to increase their physical strength and really enjoy their weight lifting. It traditionally only calls for 3 exercises – squat, deadlift and bench press, as these are the competition lifts. However, in recent years 2 common exercises have been included in the training – military press and barbell row.

I have written the exercise plans to cover all the bases so there are 2 days for each different area of the body (upper, lower and back / core). As a result, each plan has 6 days a week of training BUT you do not need to train for the full 6 days. As long as you train your body evenly (don't just focus on legs, for example), feel free to weight-train anywhere between 4 and 6 times a week, taking rest days as and when you need them. This advice is especially important with strength training – recovery is key for this goal, so training 4 days a week is enough.

Try not to train the same body part 2 days in a row, as you want to make sure each muscle group has at least 24 hours to recover after training.

You will notice that some of the exercises in the Beginner Plan start off unweighted – this is to ensure you have time to practise your form *before* you move on to lifting weights.

You'll also notice that you start on small weights, e.g. dumbbells and kettlebells, and graduate on to bigger machines, like the Smith Machine, the Squat Rack and Cables, as the weeks pass. This is deliberate and means you aren't tackling complicated equipment before you are comfortable with your weight training.

Lastly, there are many exercise repetitions in the Beginner Plan... While big compound exercises, such as squats and deadlifts, should be a weekly staple of *any* weight-lifting plan (in my opinion), the repetition of other exercises will give you time to practise and improve your lifting technique. Don't worry, every area of your body will be trained well and trained evenly, but I want you to practise training *properly* first and foremost.

When I instruct a *Comfortable Weight*, I mean a weight that challenges you but that you can lift with ease.

When I instruct a *Heavy Weight*, I mean a weight that challenges you to really push HARD by your last few reps.

You can repeat this plan for as many weeks / months as you wish. However, at some point, it would be good to progress to the Intermediate Plan...

Week 1 Form Focused
(bodyweight or comfortable weights only)

Monday + Thursday = Lower Body

Tuesday + Friday = Upper Body

Wednesday + Saturday = Back/Core

Sunday = Rest day

You'll see this is a 6-day weight-lifting plan. However, you only need to train for 4 or 5 days a week, if you'd prefer.

As long as you make sure you train your body evenly – at least 1 day on your Lower Body, 1 day on your Upper Body and 1 day on your Back/Core – feel free to weight-train anywhere between 4 and 6 days a week, taking rest days as and when you need them.

Key to symbols

 Endurance

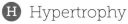 Hypertrophy

S Strength. If Strength is your goal but the symbol is missing from an exercise, leave the exercise out.

Monday + Thursday Lower Body

Squats Unweighted

Stand up straight with your feet hip-width apart. Extend your arms directly out in front of you and place one hand on top of the other – or place your hands on your hips. Keeping your back straight, lower yourself down into a deep squat by bending your hips, then knees. Pushing your weight down against your heels, stand back up straight again. Make sure your knees stay directly above your toes – they shouldn't be collapsing inward. Repeat this movement for the full amount of sets and reps.

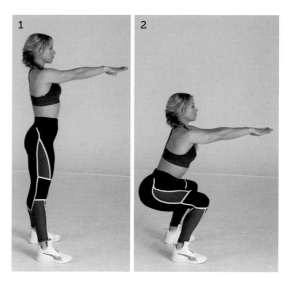

E 3 sets » 15 reps » 1 minute rest between sets

H 4 sets » 12 reps » 1 minute rest between sets

S 5 sets » 5 reps » 1 minute rest between sets

Bulgarian Split Squats on Bench Unweighted

Place a bench about 0.5m behind you. Carefully place one of your feet up on the bench behind you, resting top down. Make sure the toes of your standing foot are pointing forwards. Standing up straight and bending only at the hip and knee, come down into a low squat before pushing back up through your heel to a standing position. Repeat this movement for the full amount of sets and reps on each leg.

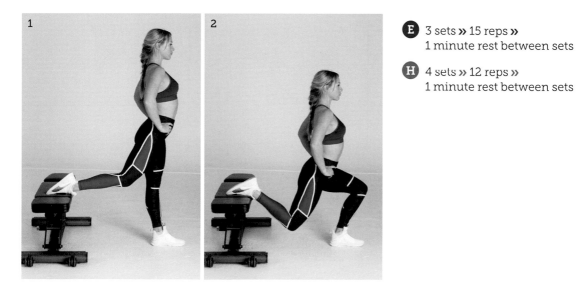

E 3 sets » 15 reps » 1 minute rest between sets

H 4 sets » 12 reps » 1 minute rest between sets

Monday + Thursday Lower Body

Hip Thrusts on Mat
Unweighted

Lie on your back with your feet hip-width apart and your knees bent. Slowly and gently raise your hips up into the air, squeezing your buttocks as you do so. Hold this position for a few seconds before slowly and gently coming back down to your starting position. Repeat this movement for the full amount of sets and reps.

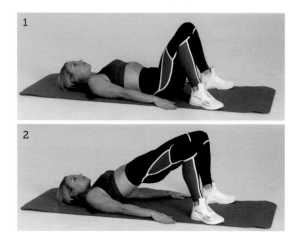

E 3 sets » 15 reps » 1 minute rest between sets

H 4 sets » 12 reps » 1 minute rest between sets

Deadlift with Olympic Bar
Unweighted

Place the bar in front of your feet. Stand up straight with your feet hip-width apart, toes pointing forwards. Keeping your back straight and bending only at the hips and knees, crouch down so your hands are able to reach the bar. Grasp the bar either side of your legs, placing one hand in an overhand grip and the other in an underhand grip (whichever is more comfortable is fine). Once you have a good grip, stand up straight, pushing down through your heels as you do so. As you come into a fully vertical standing position, squeeze your buttocks at the top of the movement. Keeping the bar against your legs, slowly allow it to pull you back down to the ground again, keeping your back straight and bending only at the hips and knees at all times. Allow the bar to hit the floor, take a breath and repeat the lift for the full amount of sets and reps.

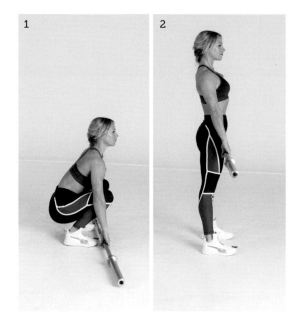

E 3 sets » 15 reps » 1 minute rest between sets

H 4 sets » 12 reps » 1 minute rest between sets

S 5 sets » 5 reps » 1 minute rest between sets

Romanian Deadlift with Olympic Bar Unweighted

Place the Olympic bar in front of your feet. Stand up straight with your feet hip-width apart and your toes pointing forwards. Keeping your back straight and bending only at the hips and knees, crouch down to grasp the bar. Grasp it either side of your legs, placing one hand in an overhand grip, the other in an underhand grip (whichever hand is more comfortable). Stand up straight, pushing down through your heels as you do so. As you come into a full standing position, squeeze your buttocks at the top of the movement. Pull your shoulders back and keep them back during the exercise. Engage your core and make sure to keep your entire core and back position solid throughout. Keeping the bar against your legs, slowly allow it to pull you down from the hips as far as your hamstrings will allow – sticking your bottom out as you go. Take a breath and return to your starting position. Repeat the lift for the full amount of sets and reps.

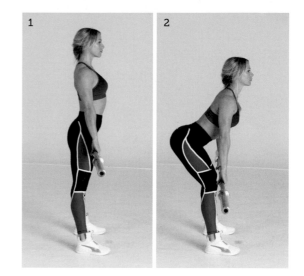

E 3 sets » 15 reps » 1 minute rest between sets

H 4 sets » 12 reps » 1 minute rest between sets

Leg Press on Machine
Comfortable weight

Sit down and place your feet hip-width apart on the plate in front of you (or slightly further apart if that is more comfortable). Point your toes upwards, or slightly outwards. Pushing through the flats of your feet, slowly and gently push against the plate. Depending on the machine, the force will either push the plate away from your seat, or your seat away from the plate. When you have fully extended (without locking your knees out – you should always keep a slight bend in them when performing a lower body lift), slowly come back into your starting position. Take a breath and repeat this movement for the full amount of sets and reps. Finish with light calf presses to exhaust. (Lower your feet to the bottom of the plate and push on to the balls of your feet. Flex your foot so your heels come back down again, then repeat to exhaust.)

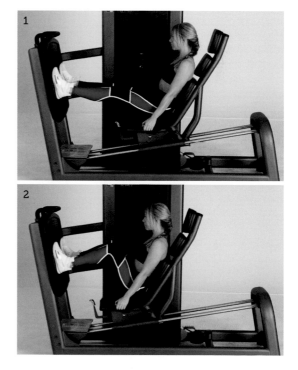

E 3 sets » 15 reps » 1 minute rest between sets

H 4 sets » 12 reps » 1 minute rest between sets

Tuesday + Friday Upper Body

Seated Dumbbell Press
Comfortable dumbbells

Adjust the bench so it's upright then sit up straight on the bench with your back against it. Hold a dumbbell in each hand and rest them on top of your thighs if need be. Bring them up to shoulder height and hold them horizontally. Push both dumbbells up into the air and gently touch them together at the top of the movement. Slowly bring them back down to shoulder height and repeat the movement for the full sets and reps.

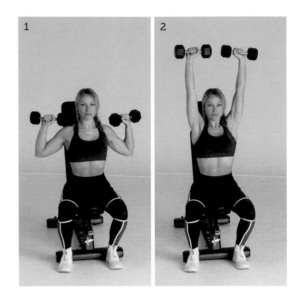

E 3 sets » 15 reps » 1 minute rest between sets

H 4 sets » 12 reps » 1 minute rest between sets

S 5 sets » 5 reps » 1 minute rest between sets

Lateral Raises
Comfortable dumbbells

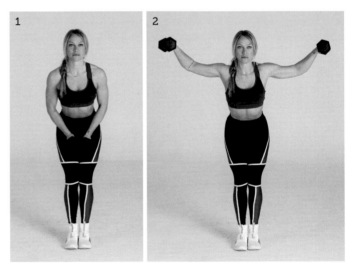

Make sure the weight is the same in each hand. Stand up straight with your knees slightly bent, your feet together. Grip the dumbbells in front of your crotch, lightly touching each other. Lean ever-so-slightly forward with your upper body, keeping a slight arch in your lower back. Keeping a slight bend in your elbows and bowing them outwards slightly, slowly and gradually raise the dumbbells out either side of you, until your arms are horizontal, like an eagle in flight. Hold this position for a fraction of a second, then slowly bring your arms back down to your starting position. Take a breath and repeat this movement for the full amount of sets and reps.

E 3 sets » 15 reps » 1 minute rest between sets

H 4 sets » 12 reps » 1 minute rest between sets

Front Raises
Comfortable dumbbells

Make sure the weight is the same in each hand. Stand up straight with your feet hip-width apart and your toes pointing forwards. Grip the dumbbells horizontally, using an overhand grip, and allow them to hang together in front of your crotch. Keeping your back straight at all times, take a deep breath and slowly raise one of the dumbbells. Keep a slight bend in your elbow as you do so. Hold the dumbbell in its raised position for a fraction of a second, then slowly bring it back down. Repeat with the other arm. Continue this movement alternately for the full amount of sets and reps.

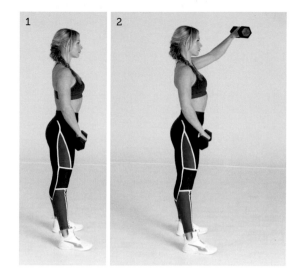

E 3 sets » 15 reps » 1 minute rest between sets

H 4 sets » 12 reps » 1 minute rest between sets

Bent Over Rows on Bench
Comfortable dumbbell

Place a dumbbell on the floor on the right-hand side of a bench. Keeping your right foot on the ground and your toes pointing forwards, place your left knee in the centre of the bench, then bend over and grip the top of the bench with your left hand. Keeping your back straight, slowly pick up the dumbbell with your right hand, making sure to keep your arm in tight to your body as you do so. Pull the dumbbell up into your armpit region and hold the dumbbell there for a fraction of a second, then slowly bring it back down to extend your arm. Continue this movement for the full amount of sets and reps, then repeat with other arm.

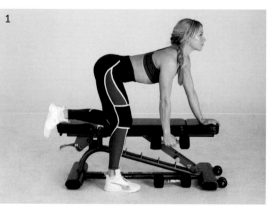

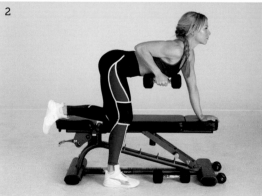

E 3 sets » 15 reps » 1 minute rest between sets

H 4 sets » 12 reps » 1 minute rest between sets

S 5 sets » 5 reps » 1 minute rest between sets

Tuesday + Friday Upper Body

Chest Press on Bench
Comfortable dumbbells

Make sure the weight is the same in each hand. Sit on the bench with your feet flat on the floor on either side and grip the dumbbells in your hands, resting them on your thighs. Lie down on the bench and pull the dumbbells up so they are just above either side of your chest, making sure they are now horizontal. Slowly push the dumbbells up until your arms are fully extended, bringing them together at the peak of the lift so they lightly touch. Slowly bring the dumbbells back down to the starting position. Take a breath and repeat this movement for the full amount of sets and reps.

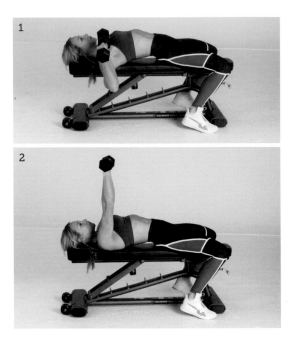

E 3 sets » 15 reps » 1 minute rest between sets

H 4 sets » 12 reps » 1 minute rest between sets

S 5 sets » 5 reps » 1 minute rest between sets

Chest Fly on Bench
Comfortable dumbbells

Make sure the weight is the same in each hand. Sit on the bench with your feet flat on the floor on either side and grip the dumbbells in your hands, resting them on top of your thighs. Lie down on the bench. Extend your arms out either side of your body at chest height. Then, as if you are hugging a beach ball, and keeping a slight bend in your elbows, bring the dumbbells together above your body. Slowly bring the dumbbells back down to the starting position. Take a breath and repeat this movement for the full amount of sets and reps.

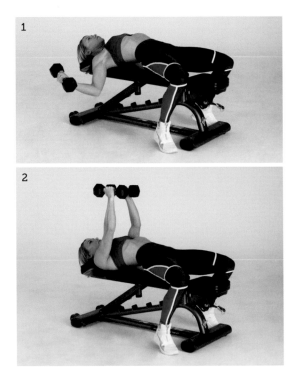

E 3 sets » 15 reps » 1 minute rest between sets

H 4 sets » 12 reps » 1 minute rest between sets

Wednesday + Saturday Back/Core

Hyperextensions Unweighted

Lie face down on the mat with your legs together. Place your hands either side of your head and slowly bow your body back into a lower back crunch (another name for this exercise is a reverse sit up). Make sure you engage your glutes and core while doing this exercise. Hold this position for a few seconds then repeat this movement for the full amount of sets and reps.

E 3 sets » 15 reps » 1 minute rest between sets

H 4 sets » 12 reps » 1 minute rest between sets

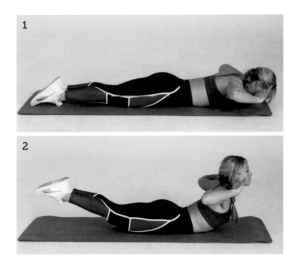

Dumbbell Pullovers on Bench
Comfortable dumbbell

Sit on the bench, legs either side of it, and grip the dumbbell (vertically) between your legs. Lie down and, as you do so, raise the dumbbell up in the air, directly above your face. Now adjust your grip by opening your hands, allowing the weight of the dumbbell to rest against the flats of your palms, gripping around its base with your fingers. Allow the dumbbell to slowly and gently come behind you, so that it is behind your head and behind the bench. Slowly and gently bring it back up into the air, above your face, into your starting position. Take a deep breath and repeat this movement for the full amount of sets and reps.

E 3 sets » 15 reps » 1 minute rest between sets

H 4 sets » 12 reps » 1 minute rest between sets

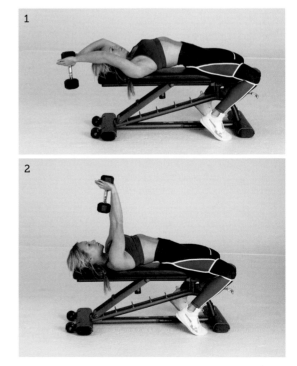

Wednesday + Saturday Back/Core

Wide Grip Rows on Machine
Comfortable weight

You can do these on a static machine or using the cable machine (as illustrated), depending on what equipment your gym has. Either sit with your legs either side of the machine or stand with your feet together and knees bent. Holding the bar using an overhand grip, take a deep breath and slowly and gently pull the bar into your chest. Hold it against yourself for a second, then slowly and gently let it pull you back to the starting position. Take a deep breath and repeat this movement for the full amount of sets and reps.

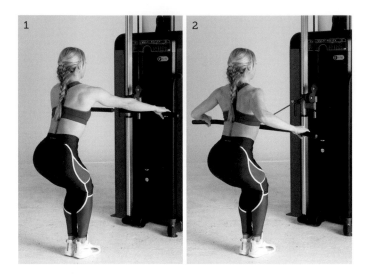

E 3 sets » 15 reps » 1 minute rest between sets

H 4 sets » 12 reps » 1 minute rest between sets

Close Grip Rows on Machine
Comfortable weight

You can do these on a static machine (as illustrated) or using the cable machine, depending on what equipment your gym has. Sit down with your legs either side of the machine and grip the handles in front of you with an inverted grip. Take a deep breath and, slowly and gently, pull the handles into your chest. Hold the handles against yourself for a second, then slowly and gently let them pull you back to the starting position. Take a deep breath and repeat this movement for the full amount of sets and reps.

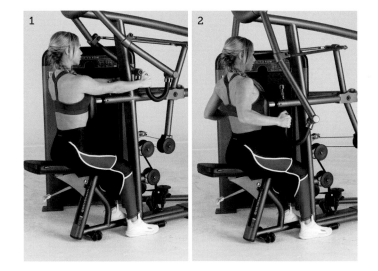

E 3 sets » 15 reps » 1 minute rest between sets

H 4 sets » 12 reps » 1 minute rest between sets

Wide Grip Pullups on Machine Fully assisted

Make sure the padded seat is upright. Facing the machine, grip the bars that are furthest apart using an overhand grip and place your knees on top of the padded seat. Slowly allow your body to drop down underneath the bars. Once your arms are fully extended, slowly pull yourself back up into a wide-grip pull-up position. Hold this for a second before allowing yourself to come back down to your starting position. Take a deep breath and repeat this movement for the full amount of sets and reps.

 E 3 sets » 15 reps »
1 minute rest between sets

H 4 sets » 12 reps »
1 minute rest between sets

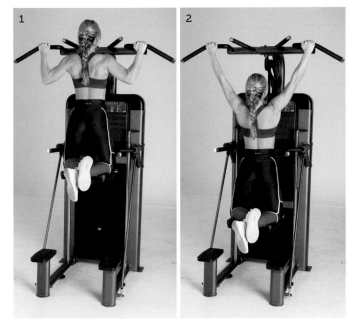

Close Grip Pullups on Machine Fully assisted

Make sure the padded seat is upright. Facing the machine, grip the bars that are closest together using an underhand grip. Place your knees on top of the seat, then slowly allow your body to drop down underneath the bars. Once your arms are fully extended, slowly pull yourself up into a pull-up position. Hold this position for a second before allowing yourself to come back down again. Take a deep breath and repeat this movement for the full amount of sets and reps.

E 3 sets » 15 reps »
1 minute rest between sets

H 4 sets » 12 reps »
1 minute rest between sets

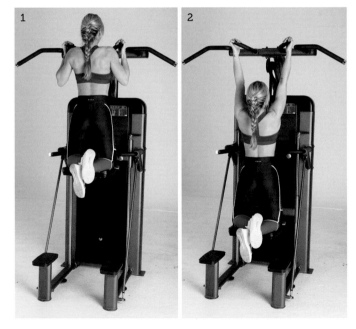

SUNDAY = FULL REST DAY

Week 2 Form with Weight Focused
(comfortable and heavy weights)

Monday + Thursday = Lower Body

Tuesday + Friday = Upper Body

Wednesday + Saturday = Back/Core

Sunday = Full Rest Day

You'll see this is a 6-day weight-lifting plan. However, you only need to train for 4 or 5 days a week, if you'd prefer.

As long as you make sure you train your body evenly – at least 1 day on your Lower Body, 1 day on your Upper Body and 1 day on your Back/Core – feel free to weight-train anywhere between 4 and 6 days a week, taking rest days as and when you need them.

Key to symbols

E Endurance

H Hypertrophy

S Strength. If Strength is your goal but the symbol is missing from an exercise, leave the exercise out.

Monday + Thursday Lower Body

Goblet Squats Comfortable kettlebell or dumbbell

Grab a kettlebell or dumbbell and hold it in front of your chest, against your body. Stand up straight with your feet hip-width apart. Keeping your back straight, lower yourself down into a deep squat by bending your hips, then knees. Pushing your weight down against your heels, stand back up straight again. Make sure your knees stay directly above your toes – they shouldn't be collapsing inward. Repeat this movement for the full amount of sets and reps.

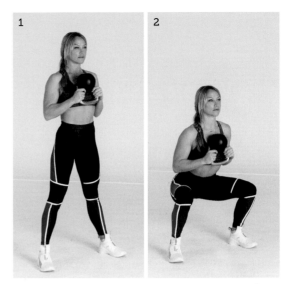

E 3 sets » 15 reps » 1 minute rest between sets

H 4 sets » 12 reps » 1 minute rest between sets

S 5 sets » 5 reps » 1 minute rest between sets

Bulgarian Split Squats on Bench
Comfortable kettlebells or dumbbells

Place a bench about 0.5m behind you. Grab two kettlebells or dumbbells of the same weight and hold one in each hand. Carefully place one of your feet up on the bench behind you, resting top down. Make sure the toes of your standing foot are pointing forwards. Standing up straight and bending only at the hip and knee, come down into a low squat before pushing back up through your heel to a standing position. Repeat this movement for the full amount of sets and reps on each leg.

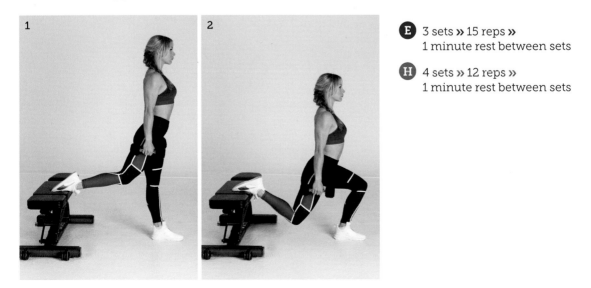

E 3 sets » 15 reps » 1 minute rest between sets

H 4 sets » 12 reps » 1 minute rest between sets

Monday + Thursday Lower Body

Hip Thrusts on Mat
Comfortable kettlebell or dumbbell

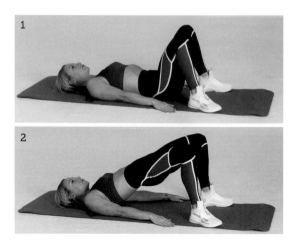

(Please note: the illustration shows the hip thrust unweighted – this exercise should be weighted.) Lie on your back with your feet hip-width apart and your knees bent. Place the weight on your crotch, or wherever is most comfortable. Holding the weight in place, slowly and gently raise your hips up into the air, squeezing your buttocks as you do so. Hold this position for a few seconds before slowly and gently coming back down to your starting position. Repeat this movement for the full amount of sets and reps.

E 3 sets » 15 reps » 1 minute rest between sets

H 4 sets » 12 reps » 1 minute rest between sets

Deadlift with Olympic Bar
Comfortable weight

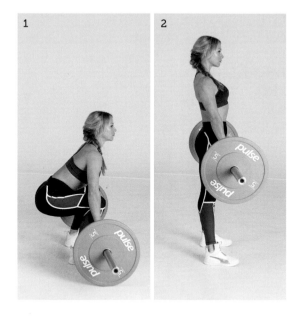

Make sure the weight is the same each side – use clips if you need to. Place the bar in front of your feet. Stand up straight with your feet hip-width apart, toes pointing forwards. Keeping your back straight and bending only at the hips and knees, crouch down so your hands are able to reach the bar. Grasp the bar either side of your legs, placing one hand in an overhand grip and the other in an underhand grip (whichever is more comfortable is fine). Once you have a good grip, stand up straight, pushing down through your heels as you do so. As you come into a fully vertical standing position, squeeze your buttocks at the top of the movement. Keeping the bar against your legs, slowly allow it to pull you back down to the ground again, keeping your back straight and bending only at the hips and knees at all times. Allow the bar to hit the floor, take a breath and repeat the lift for the full amount of sets and reps.

E 3 sets » 15 reps » 1 minute rest between sets

H 4 sets » 12 reps » 1 minute rest between sets

S 5 sets » 5 reps » 1 minute rest between sets

Romanian Deadlift with Olympic Bar Comfortable weight

Make sure the weight is the same each side – use clips if you need to. Place the bar horizontally in front of your feet. Stand up straight with your feet hip-width apart and your toes pointing forwards. Keeping your back straight and bending only at the hips and knees, crouch down to grasp the bar. Grasp it either side of your legs, placing one hand in an overhand grip, the other in an underhand grip (whichever hand is more comfortable). Stand up straight, pushing down through your heels as you do so. As you come into a full standing position, squeeze your buttocks at the top of the movement. Pull your shoulders back and keep them back during the exercise. Engage your core and make sure to keep your entire core and back position solid throughout. Keeping the bar against your legs, slowly allow it to pull you down from the hips as far as your hamstrings will allow – sticking your bottom out as you go. Take a breath and return to your starting position. Repeat the lift for the full amount of sets and reps.

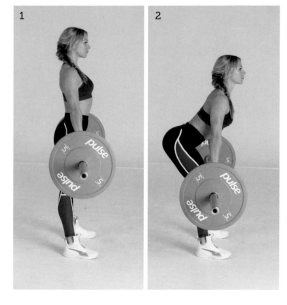

E 3 sets » 15 reps » 1 minute rest between sets

H 4 sets » 12 reps » 1 minute rest between sets

Leg Press on Machine
Heavy weight

Sit down and place your feet hip-width apart on the plate in front of you (or slightly further apart if that is more comfortable). Point your toes upwards, or slightly outwards. Pushing through the flats of your feet, slowly and gently push against the plate. Depending on the machine, the force will either push the plate away from your seat, or your seat away from the plate. When you have fully extended (without locking your knees out – you should always keep a slight bend in them when performing a lower body lift), slowly come back into your starting position. Take a breath and repeat this movement for the full amount of sets and reps. Finish with light calf presses to exhaust.

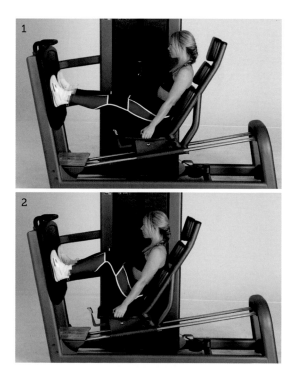

E 3 sets » 15 reps » 1 minute rest between sets

H 4 sets » 12 reps » 1 minute rest between sets

Tuesday + Friday Upper Body

Seated Military Press Comfortable barbell

Grip the bar with your hands shoulder-width apart, using an overhand grip. Resting the bar on top of your thighs, sit down on the bench, with your back fully upright against it and your feet either side. Swiftly lift the bar up so that it is at chest height then push the bar up above your head until your arms are fully extended. Hold the bar above your head for a second, then slowly bring it back down to chest height. Take a deep breath and repeat this movement for the full amount of sets and reps.

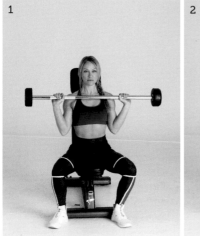
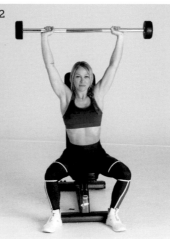

E 3 sets » 15 reps » 1 minute rest between sets

H 4 sets » 12 reps » 1 minute rest between sets

S 5 sets » 5 reps » 1 minute rest between sets

Lateral Raises
Heavy dumbbells

Make sure the weight is the same in each hand. Stand up straight with your knees slightly bent and your feet together. Grip the dumbbells in front of your crotch, lightly touching each other. Lean ever-so-slightly forward with your upper body, keeping a slight arch in your lower back. Keeping a slight bend in your elbows and bowing them outwards slightly, slowly and gradually raise the dumbbells out either side of you, until your arms are horizontal, like an eagle in flight. Hold this position for a fraction of a second, then slowly bring your arms back down to your starting position. Take a breath and repeat this movement for the full amount of sets and reps.

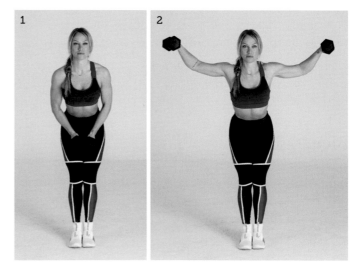

E 3 sets » 15 reps » 1 minute rest between sets

H 4 sets » 12 reps » 1 minute rest between sets

Front Raises with Weight Plate
Comfortable weight

Stand up straight with your feet hip-width apart. Grabbing the weight with both hands, hold it in front of your stomach. Extending your arms, bring the weight up in front of your chest, always keeping a slight bend in your elbows. Hold the weight for a second, then slowly bring it back down to stomach height. Take a deep breath and repeat this movement for the full amount of sets and reps.

E 3 sets » 15 reps » 1 minute rest between sets

H 4 sets » 12 reps » 1 minute rest between sets

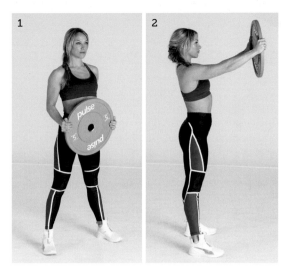

Bent Over Rows with Olympic Bar *Unweighted*

Stand up straight with your feet hip-width apart. Grab the bar with both hands and pull your shoulders back. Keeping an arch in your back and holding the bar against your lower body, slowly come down into a hamstring stretch until you have reached your full range of motion. Once there, pull the bar up into your ribcage, then slowly lower it back down again. Take a deep breath and repeat this movement for the full amount of sets and reps.

E 3 sets » 15 reps » 1 minute rest between sets

H 4 sets » 12 reps » 1 minute rest between sets

S 5 sets » 5 reps » 1 minute rest between sets

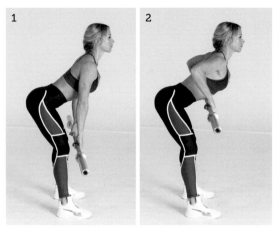

Bicep Curls
Comfortable dumbbells

Stand up straight with your feet hip-width apart. Grip a dumbbell in each hand and allow them to hang either side of your hips. Keeping your arms in tight to your sides at all times, slowly lift the dumbbells from hip height into your shoulders, twisting the dumbbells into a horizontal position as you do so. Slowly lower the dumbbells back down to their starting position. Continue this movement for the full amount of sets and reps.

E 3 sets » 15 reps » 1 minute rest between sets

H 4 sets » 12 reps » 1 minute rest between sets

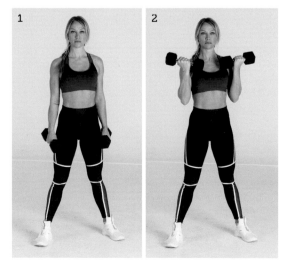

Tuesday + Friday Upper Body

Chest Press with Olympic Bar
Comfortable weight

(I would rather you use a bench press – a bench underneath a racked Olympic bar – for chest press exercies. However, if you have to use a Smith machine – illustrated here – that's fine.) Lie back on the bench with your feet either side and flat on the floor. Reaching up, grip the bar with both hands – your hands should be directly above your shoulders. Push the bar up so it is free from the holding, then bring it down slowly so it lightly touches your chest. Push the bar back up into the air and hold it there for a second before bringing it back down. Repeat this movement for the full amount of sets and reps.

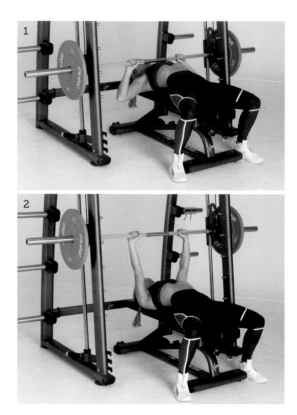

E 3 sets » 15 reps » 1 minute rest between sets

H 4 sets » 12 reps » 1 minute rest between sets

S 5 sets » 5 reps » 1 minute rest between sets

Tricep Dips on Bench Unweighted

Sit on a bench and place your hands flat on top of it, either side of your body. Extend your legs out in front of you. Push yourself slightly above and in front of the bench. Keeping your elbows in tight to your sides, slowly allow your body to drop down. When you have come down as far as possible, slowly push yourself back up, using your triceps. Take a deep breath and repeat this movement for the full amount of sets and reps.

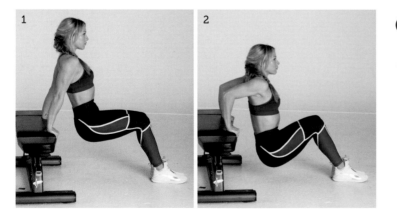

E 3 sets » 15 reps » 1 minute rest between sets

H 4 sets » 12 reps » 1 minute rest between sets

Wednesday + Saturday Back/Core

Hyperextensions Unweighted

Lie face down on the mat and place your hands either side of your head. Slowly bow your body back into a lower back crunch (another name for this exercise is a reverse sit up). Make sure you engage your glutes and core while doing this exercise. Hold this position for a few seconds then repeat this movement for the full amount of sets and reps.

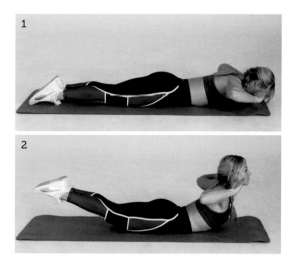

E 3 sets » 15 reps » 1 minute rest between sets

H 4 sets » 12 reps » 1 minute rest between sets

Dumbbell Pullovers on Bench
Heavy dumbbell

Sit on the bench, legs either side of it, and grip the dumbbell (vertically) between your legs. Lie down and, as you do so, raise the dumbbell up in the air, directly above your face. Now adjust your grip by opening your hands, allowing the weight of the dumbbell to rest against the flats of your palms, gripping around its base with your fingers. Allow the dumbbell to slowly and gently come behind you, so that it is behind your head and behind the bench. Slowly and gently bring it back up into the air, above your face, into your starting position. Take a deep breath and repeat this movement for the full amount of sets and reps.

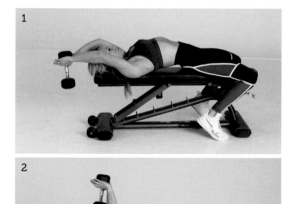

E 3 sets » 15 reps » 1 minute rest between sets

H 4 sets » 12 reps » 1 minute rest between sets

Wednesday + Saturday Back/Core

Wide Grip Rows on Machine
Heavy weight

You can do these on a static machine or using the cable machine (as illustrated), depending on what equipment your gym has. Either sit with your legs either side of the machine or stand with your feet together and knees bent. Holding the bar using an overhand grip, take a deep breath and slowly and gently pull the bar into your chest. Hold it against yourself for a second, then slowly and gently let it pull you back to the starting position. Take a deep breath and repeat this movement for the full amount of sets and reps.

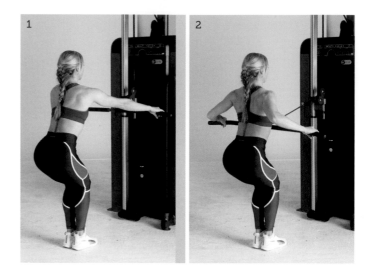

E 3 sets » 15 reps » 1 minute rest between sets

H 4 sets » 12 reps » 1 minute rest between sets

Close Grip Rows on Machine Heavy weight

You can do these on a static machine (as illustrated) or using the cable machine, depending on what equipment your gym has. Sit down with your legs either side of the machine and grip the handles in front of you with an inverted grip. Take a deep breath and, slowly and gently, pull the handles into your chest. Hold the handles against yourself for a second, then slowly and gently let them pull you back to the starting position. Take a deep breath and repeat this movement for the full amount of sets and reps.

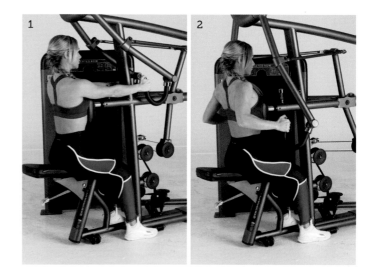

E 3 sets » 15 reps » 1 minute rest between sets

H 4 sets » 12 reps » 1 minute rest between sets

Wide Grip Pullups on Machine Fully assisted

Make sure the padded seat is upright. Facing the machine, grip the bars that are furthest apart using an overhand grip and place your knees on top of the padded seat. Slowly allow your body to drop down underneath the bars. Once your arms are fully extended, slowly pull yourself back up into a wide-grip pull-up position. Hold this for a second before allowing yourself to come back down to your starting position. Take a deep breath and repeat this movement for the full amount of sets and reps.

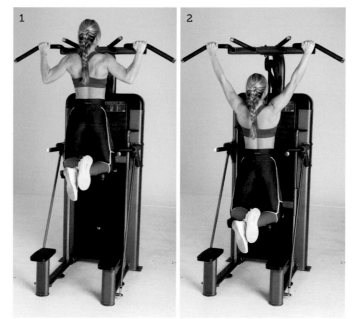

E 3 sets » 15 reps »
1 minute rest between sets

H 4 sets » 12 reps »
1 minute rest between sets

Close Grip Pullups on Machine Fully assisted

Make sure the padded seat is upright. Facing the machine, grip the bars that are closest together using an underhand grip. Place your knees on top of the seat, then slowly allow your body to drop down underneath the bars. Once your arms are fully extended, slowly pull yourself up into a pull-up position. Hold this position for a second before allowing yourself to come back down again. Take a deep breath and repeat this movement for the full amount of sets and reps.

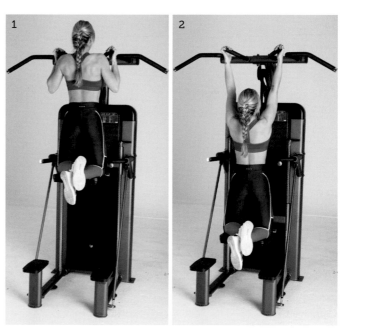

E 3 sets » 15 reps »
1 minute rest between sets

H 4 sets » 12 reps »
1 minute rest between sets

SUNDAY = FULL REST DAY

Week 3 Form and Weight Focused
(comfortable and heavy weights)

Monday + Thursday = Lower Body

Tuesday + Friday = Upper Body

Wednesday + Saturday = Back/Core

Sunday = Full Rest Day

You'll see this is a 6-day weight-lifting plan. However, you only need to train for 4 or 5 days a week, if you'd prefer.

As long as you make sure you train your body evenly – at least 1 day on your Lower Body, 1 day on your Upper Body and 1 day on your Back/Core – feel free to weight-train anywhere between 4 and 6 days a week, taking rest days as and when you need them.

Key to symbols

E Endurance

H Hypertrophy

S Strength. If Strength is your goal but the symbol is missing from an exercise, leave the exercise out.

Monday + Thursday Lower Body

Squats on Smith Machine Comfortable weight

Make sure the weight is the same on each side. Find the centre of the horizontal bar and duck underneath it, so the bar is resting across your shoulders. Place your feet hip-width apart, or slightly further if that is more comfortable, and make sure your toes are either pointing forwards or slightly outwards. Take hold of the bar either side of your shoulders and unhook it from the machine – keep it unhooked using your grip. Standing up straight and bending only at the hips and knees, come down into a low squat before pushing back up through your heels to a standing position, squeezing your glutes as you do so. Take a breath and repeat this movement for the full amount of sets and reps.

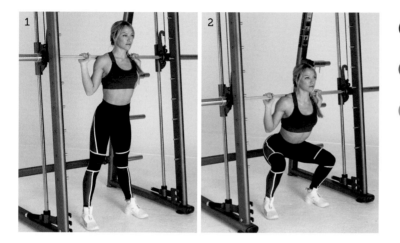

E 3 sets » 15 reps »
1 minute rest between sets

H 4 sets » 12 reps »
1 minute rest between sets

S 5 sets » 5 reps »
1 minute rest between sets

Bulgarian Split Squats on Smith Machine Comfortable weight

Place the bench about 0.5m behind you. Find the centre of the horizontal bar and duck underneath it, so the bar is resting across your shoulders. Place one foot up on the bench behind you, resting top down. Make sure the toes of your standing foot are pointing forwards. Take hold of the bar either side of your shoulders and unhook the bar from the machine – keep it unhooked using your grip. Standing up straight and bending only at the hip and knee, come down into a low squat before pushing back up through your heel to a standing position. Take a breath and repeat on the other leg. Repeat for the full amount of sets and reps.

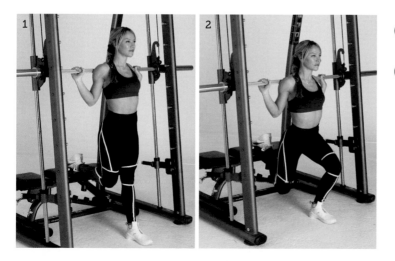

E 3 sets » 15 reps »
1 minute rest between sets

H 4 sets » 12 reps »
1 minute rest between sets

Monday + Thursday Lower Body

Hip Thrusts on Smith Machine Comfortable weight

(Please note: the illustration shows the Smith unweighted – this exercise should be weighted.)
Place the bench about 0.5m behind you, so you are sandwiched between the Smith and the bench.
Lower the bar so it is about 30cm off the ground. Sit down on the floor between the bar and the
bench, resting your upper back and shoulder blades on the edge of the bench. Place a bar pad (a black,
cushioned tube) around the centre of the horizontal bar. Place your feet hip-width apart and keep your
toes pointing forwards or slightly outwards. Place your hips underneath the cushion and your hands
either side of your hips. Unhook the bar from the machine – keep it unhooked using your grip – and
thrust up into the air, through your glutes, squeezing them tight at the top of the movement. Hold this
position for a few seconds before coming back down until your buttocks are just above the ground.
Take a breath and repeat this movement for the full amount of sets and reps.

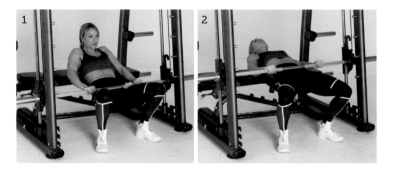

E 3 sets » 15 reps »
1 minute rest between sets

H 4 sets » 12 reps »
1 minute rest between sets

Deadlift with Olympic Bar
Heavy weight

Make sure the weight is the same each side – use
clips if you need to. Place the bar in front of your
feet. Stand up straight with your feet hip-width
apart, toes pointing forwards. Keeping your back
straight and bending only at the hips and knees,
crouch down so your hands are able to reach the
bar. Grasp the bar either side of your legs, placing
one hand in an overhand grip and the other in an
underhand grip (whichever is more comfortable
is fine). Once you have a good grip, stand up
straight, pushing down through your heels as
you do so. As you come into a fully vertical
standing position, squeeze your buttocks at the
top of the movement. Keeping the bar against
your legs, slowly allow it to pull you back down to
the ground again, keeping your back straight and
bending only at the hips and knees at all times.
Allow the bar to hit the floor, take a breath and
repeat the lift for the full amount of sets and reps.

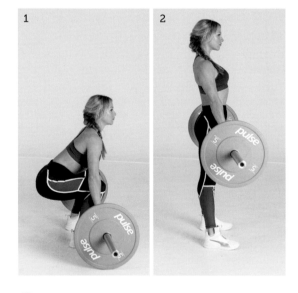

E 3 sets » 15 reps » 1 minute rest between sets

H 4 sets » 12 reps » 1 minute rest between sets

S 5 sets » 5 reps » 3 minute rest between sets

Romanian Deadlift with Olympic Bar Heavy weight

Make sure the weight is the same each side – use clips if you need to. Place the bar horizontally in front of your feet. Stand up straight with your feet hip-width apart and your toes pointing forwards. Keeping your back straight and bending only at the hips and knees, crouch down to grasp the bar. Grasp it either side of your legs, placing one hand in an overhand grip, the other in an underhand grip (whichever hand is more comfortable). Stand up straight, pushing down through your heels as you do so. As you come into a full standing position, squeeze your buttocks at the top of the movement. Pull your shoulders back and keep them back during the exercise. Engage your core and make sure to keep your entire core and back position solid throughout. Keeping the bar against your legs, slowly allow it to pull you down from the hips as far as your hamstrings will allow – sticking your bottom out as you go. Take a breath and return to your starting position. Repeat the lift for the full amount of sets and reps.

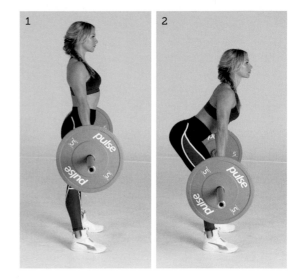

E 3 sets » 15 reps » 1 minute rest between sets

H 4 sets » 12 reps » 1 minute rest between sets

Leg Press on Machine Heavy weight

Sit down and place your feet hip-width apart on the plate in front of you (or slightly further apart if that is more comfortable). Point your toes upwards, or slightly outwards. Pushing through the flats of your feet, slowly and gently push against the plate. Depending on the machine, the force will either push the plate away from your seat, or your seat away from the plate. When you have fully extended (without locking your knees out – you should always keep a slight bend in them when performing a lower body lift), slowly come back into your starting position. Take a breath and repeat this movement for the full amount of sets and reps. Finish with light calf presses to exhaust.

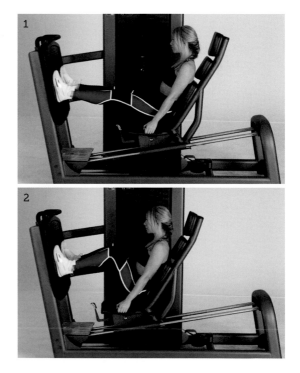

E 3 sets » 15 reps » 1 minute rest between sets.

H 4 sets » 12 reps » 1 minute rest between sets.

Tuesday + Friday Upper Body

Shoulder Press on Smith Machine Comfortable weight

Sit down and grab the bar with both hands in an overhand grip. Push the bar up into the air and hold it there for a second before slowly bringing it back down. Repeat this movement for the full amount of sets and reps.

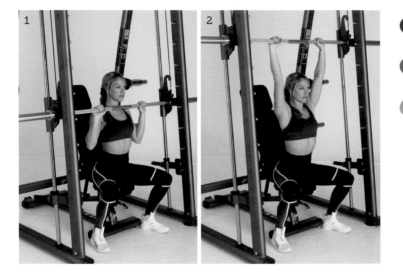

E 3 sets » 15 reps »
1 minute rest between sets

H 4 sets » 12 reps »
1 minute rest between sets

S 5 sets » 5 reps »
1 minute rest between sets

Lateral Raises on Cable Machine
Comfortable weight

Attach the correct handle to the cable and make sure the weight you choose on the machine is very light (shoulders only need a light weight). With a slight bend in your elbow, and keeping your arm locked in this position, slowly raise the handle into the air until your arm is horizontal. Allow the handle to pull your arm slowly back down into your starting position. Repeat this movement for the full amount of sets and reps on each arm.

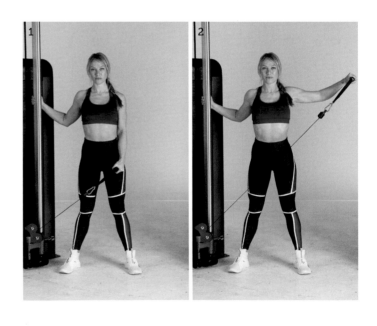

E 3 sets » 15 reps »
1 minute rest between sets

H 4 sets » 12 reps »
1 minute rest between sets

Front Raises on Cable Machine
Comfortable weight

Attach the correct handle to the cable and make sure the weight you choose on the machine is very light (shoulders only need a light weight). With a slight bend in your elbows, and keeping your arms locked in this position, slowly raise the handle up into the air out in front of you. Allow the handle to slowly pull your arms back down into your starting position. Repeat this movement for the full amount of sets and reps on each arm.

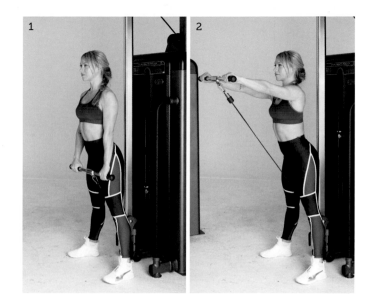

(E) 3 sets » 15 reps » 1 minute rest between sets

(H) 4 sets » 12 reps » 1 minute rest between sets

Bent Over Rows on Bench
Heavy dumbbell

Place a dumbbell on the floor on the right-hand side of a bench. Keeping your right foot on the ground and your toes pointing forwards, place your left knee in the centre of the bench, then bend over and grip the top of the bench with your left hand. Keeping your back straight, slowly pick up the dumbbell with your right hand, making sure to keep your arm in tight to your body as you do so. Pull the dumbbell up into your armpit region and hold the dumbbell there for a fraction of a second, then slowly bring it back down to extend your arm. Continue this movement for the full amount of sets and reps, then repeat with the other arm.

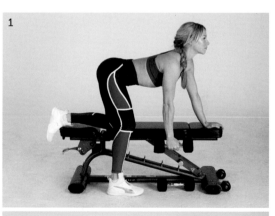

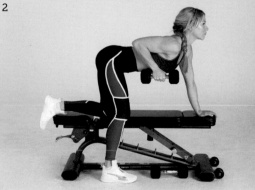

(E) 3 sets » 15 reps » 1 minute rest between sets

(H) 4 sets » 12 reps » 1 minute rest between sets

(S) 5 sets » 5 reps » 3 minutes rest between sets

Tuesday + Friday Upper Body

Chest Press with Olympic Bar Comfortable weight

(I would rather you use a bench press – a bench underneath a racked Olympic bar – for chest press exercises. However, if you have to use a Smith machine – illustrated here – that's fine.) Make sure the weight is the same each side. Lie back on the bench with your feet either side and flat on the floor. Reaching up, grip the bar with both hands – your hands should be directly above your shoulders. Push the bar up so it is free from the holding, then bring it down slowly so it lightly touches your chest. Push the bar back up into the air and hold it there for a second before bringing it back down. Repeat this movement for the full amount of sets and reps.

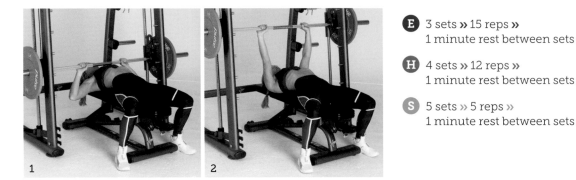

1   2

E 3 sets » 15 reps »
1 minute rest between sets

H 4 sets » 12 reps »
1 minute rest between sets

S 5 sets » 5 reps »
1 minute rest between sets

Chest Fly on Cable Machine Comfortable weight

You will need a cable machine with two columns. Place the correct handles on both of the cables, and make sure you choose the same weight on each side. Raise the handles so they are slightly above shoulder height – make sure they are the same height on each side. Grab one cable with one hand and then reach over and grab the other. Holding a handle in each hand, take a big step forward with one leg – like a lunge but not as deep. Keep a slight bend in both elbows and pull both cables together, out in front of your chest, as if you are hugging a beach ball. Allow the cables to pull you slowly and gently back into your starting position. Repeat this movement for the full amount of sets and reps.

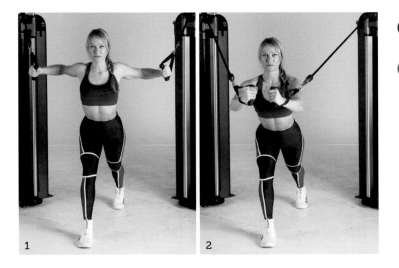

1   2

E 3 sets » 15 reps »
1 minute rest between sets

H 4 sets » 12 reps »
1 minute rest between sets

Wednesday + Saturday Back/Core

Leg Raises on Machine Unweighted

Stand on the leg raise machine. Keep your back straight against the back pad and grip both the handles. Let your legs dangle underneath you and cross your ankles. Slowly raise your legs up in front of you, then slowly allow them to come back down to your starting position. Repeat this movement fluidly to exhaust.

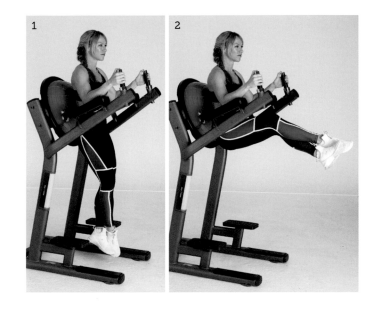

E 1 set to exhaust

H 1 set to exhaust

Elbows to Hand Plank
Unweighted

You may need a mat or cushion for your elbows during this exercise. Lie on your front with your feet hip-width apart, resting your toes against the mat. Lean on your elbows and keep your forearms flat against the mat. Make sure your elbows are underneath your shoulders. Pushing against your toes and forearms, raise your upper body into the air, one arm at a time, to rest on your hands, so you form an elevated plank. Do not allow your spine to curve, either concavely or convexly. You want a straight back. Come back down to rest on your forearms, one arm at a time, and then push back up on to your hands. Repeat to exhaust.

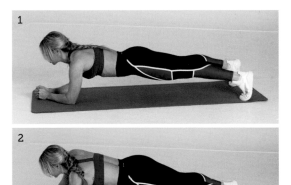

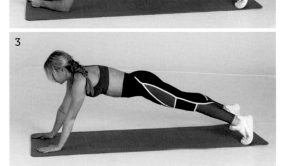

E 1 set to exhaust

H 1 set to exhaust

Wednesday + Saturday Back/Core

Single Arm Alternate Wide Grip Rows Comfortable weight

Sit down with your legs either side of the machine and grip one of the handles in front of you, with an overhand grip. Take a deep breath, then slowly and gently pull the handle into your chest. Hold the handle against yourself for a second, then slowly and gently let it pull you back to the starting position. Take a deep breath and repeat this movement for the full amount of reps on each arm.

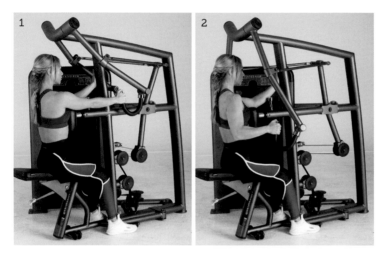

E 3 sets » 15 reps »
1 minute rest between sets

H 4 sets » 12 reps »
1 minute rest between sets

Single Arm Alternate Close Grip Rows Comfortable weight

You can do these sitting on the floor in front of the cable machine or standing, whichever you prefer. I like to do the exercises standing when I can, as per the illustration. Grip one handle with an inverted grip, take a deep breath then slowly and gently pull the handle into your chest. Hold the handle against yourself for a second, then slowly and gently let it pull you back to the starting position. Take a deep breath and repeat this movement for the full amount of reps, on each arm.

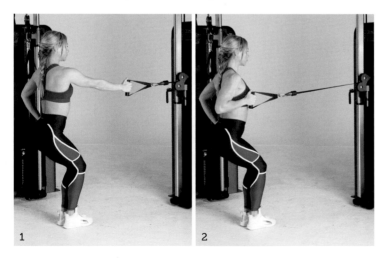

E 3 sets » 15 reps »
1 minute rest between sets

H 4 sets » 12 reps »
1 minute rest between sets

Wide Grip Pulldowns on Cable Machine
Comfortable weight

You can do this on a specific cable machine with a bench attached, or you can improvise as I have done in the illustration, by pulling a bench up close to any cable machine. Attach the long bar to the cable machine and make sure it's at its highest setting. Sit down on the bench, fully upright, and grab the bar on either side of the cable with an overhand grip. Pull the bar down in front of your chest and slowly let it pull your arms back up again. Repeat this movement for the full amount of sets and reps.

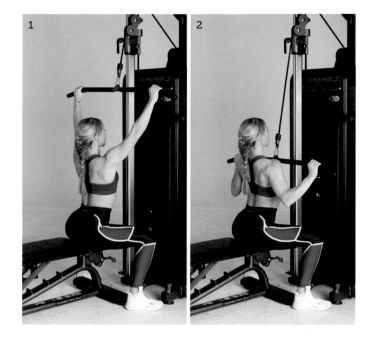

 3 sets » 15 reps »
1 minute rest between sets

 4 sets » 12 reps »
1 minute rest between sets

Close Grip Pulldowns on Cable Machine
Comfortable weight

You can do this on a specific cable machine with a bench attached, or you can improvise, as I have done in the illustration, by pulling a bench up close to any cable machine. Attach any bar to the cable machine and make sure it's at its highest setting. Sit down on the bench, fully upright, and grab the bar on either side of the cable with an underhand grip. Pull the bar down in front of your chest and slowly let it pull your arms back up again. Repeat this movement for the full amount of sets and reps.

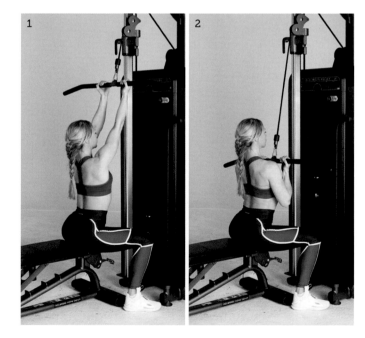

 3 sets » 15 reps »
1 minute rest between sets

 4 sets » 12 rep »
1 minute rest between sets

SUNDAY = FULL REST DAY

Beginner

> **Week 4** Form and Weight Focused
> *(comfortable and heavy weights)*
>
> Monday + Thursday = Lower Body
>
> Tuesday + Friday = Upper Body
>
> Wednesday + Saturday = Back/Core
>
> Sunday = Full Rest Day

You'll see this is a 6-day weight-lifting plan. However, you only need to train for 4 or 5 days a week, if you'd prefer.

As long as you make sure you train your body evenly – at least 1 day on your Lower Body, 1 day on your Upper Body and 1 day on your Back/Core – feel free to weight-train anywhere between 4 and 6 days a week, taking rest days as and when you need them.

Key to symbols

 Endurance

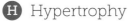 Hypertrophy

S Strength. If Strength is your goal but the symbol is missing from an exercise, leave the exercise out.

Monday + Thursday Lower Body

Squats on Squat Rack with Olympic Bar Unweighted

Find the centre of the horizontal bar and duck underneath it, so the bar is resting across your shoulders. Take hold of the bar either side of your shoulders and come up slightly on your tiptoes. Remove the bar from its holdings and take a few cautious steps backwards. Place your feet hip-width apart, or slightly further if that is a more comfortable squat position for you, and make sure your toes are either pointing forwards or slightly outwards, whichever is more comfortable. Standing up straight and bending only at the hip and knees, come down into a low squat before pushing back up through your heels to a standing position, squeezing your glutes as you do so. Take a breath and repeat this movement for the full amount of sets and reps.

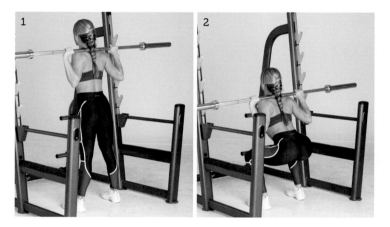

E 3 sets » 15 reps »
1 minute rest between sets

H 4 sets » 12 reps »
1 minute rest between sets

S 5 sets » 5 reps »
1 minute rest between sets

Bulgarian Split Squat on Smith Machine Heavy weight

(Please note: the illustration shows the Smith unweighted – this exercise should be weighted.) Make sure the weight is the same on each side. Place the bench about 0.5m behind you. Find the centre of the horizontal bar and duck underneath it, so the bar is resting across your shoulders. Place one foot up on the bench behind you, resting top down. Make sure the toes of your standing foot are pointing forwards. Take hold of the bar either side of your shoulders and unhook the bar from the machine – keep it unhooked using your grip. Standing up straight and bending only at the hip and knee, come down into a low squat before pushing back up through your heel to a standing position. Take a breath and repeat on the other leg. Repeat this movement for the full amount of sets and reps.

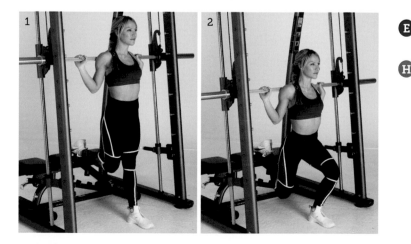

E 3 sets » 15 reps »
1 minute rest between sets

H 4 sets » 12 reps »
1 minute rest between sets

Monday + Thursday Lower Body

Hip Thrusts on Smith Machine Heavy weight

(Please note: the illustration shows the Smith unweighted – this exercise should be weighted.)
Place the bench about 0.5m behind you, so you are sandwiched between the Smith and the bench.
Lower the bar so it is about 30cm off the ground. Sit down on the floor between the bar and the bench,
facing the bar and resting your upper back and shoulder blades on the edge of the bench. Place a bar
pad (a black, cushioned tube) around the centre of the horizontal bar. Place your feet hip-width apart
and keep your toes pointing forwards or slightly outwards. Place your hips underneath the cushion
and your hands either side of your hips. Unhook the bar from the machine – keep it unhooked using
your grip – and thrust up into the air, through your glutes, squeezing them tight at the top of the
movement. Hold this position for a few seconds before coming back down until your buttocks are
just above the ground. Take a breath and repeat this movement for the full amount of sets and reps.

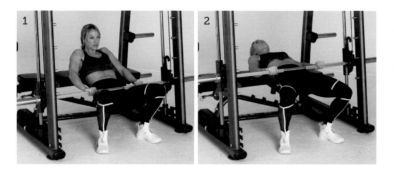

E 3 sets » 15 reps »
1 minute rest between sets

H 4 sets » 12 reps »
1 minute rest between sets

Deadlift with Olympic Bar
Heavy weight

Make sure the weight is the same each side – use
clips if you need to. Place the bar in front of your
feet. Stand up straight with your feet hip-width
apart, toes pointing forwards. Keeping your back
straight and bending only at the hips and knees,
crouch down so your hands are able to reach the
bar. Grasp the bar either side of your legs, placing
one hand in an overhand grip and the other in an
underhand grip (whichever is more comfortable
is fine). Once you have a good grip, stand up
straight, pushing down through your heels as
you do so. As you come into a fully vertical
standing position, squeeze your buttocks at the
top of the movement. Keeping the bar against
your legs, slowly allow it to pull you back down
to the ground again, keeping your back straight
and bending only at the hips and knees at all times.
Allow the bar to hit the floor, take a breath and
repeat the lift for the full amount of sets and reps.

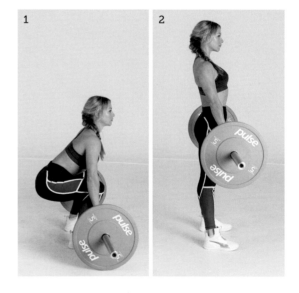

E 3 sets » 15 reps » 1 minute rest between sets

H 4 sets » 12 reps » 1 minute rest between sets

S 5 sets » 5 reps » 3 minute rest between sets

Romanian Deadlift with Olympic Bar Heavy weight

Make sure the weight is the same on each side – use clips if you need to. Place the bar horizontally in front of your feet. Stand up straight with your feet hip-width apart and your toes pointing forwards. Keeping your back straight and bending only at the hips and knees, crouch down to grasp the bar. Grasp it either side of your legs, placing one hand in an overhand grip, the other in an underhand grip (whichever hand is more comfortable). Stand up straight, pushing down through your heels as you do so. As you come into a full standing position, squeeze your buttocks at the top of the movement. Pull your shoulders back and keep them back during the exercise. Engage your core and make sure to keep your entire core and back position solid throughout. Keeping the bar against your legs, slowly allow it to pull you down from the hips as far as your hamstrings will allow – sticking your bottom out as you go. Take a breath and return to your starting position. Repeat the lift for the full amount of sets and reps.

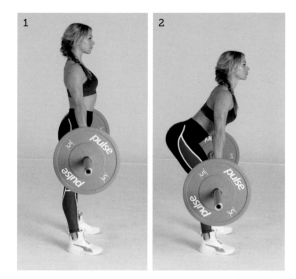

E 3 sets » 15 reps » 1 minute rest between sets

H 4 sets » 12 reps » 1 minute rest between sets

Leg Press on Machine Heavy weight

Sit down and place your feet hip-width apart on the plate in front of you (or slightly further apart if that is more comfortable). Point your toes upwards, or slightly outwards. Pushing through the flats of your feet, slowly and gently push against the plate. Depending on the machine, the force will either push the plate away from your seat, or your seat away from the plate. When you have fully extended (without locking your knees out – you should always keep a slight bend in them when performing a lower body lift), slowly come back into your starting position. Take a breath and repeat this movement for the full amount of sets and reps. Finish with light calf presses to exhaust.

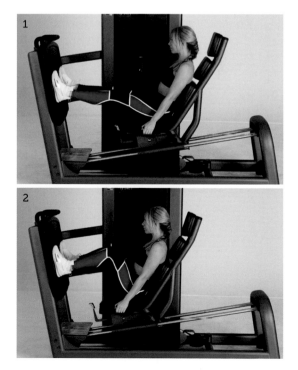

E 3 sets » 15 reps » 1 minute rest between sets

H 4 sets » 12 reps » 1 minute rest between sets

Tuesday + Friday Upper Body

Seated Dumbbell Press
Heavy dumbbells

Adjust the bench so it's upright then sit up straight on the bench with your back against it. Hold a dumbbell in each hand and rest them on top of your thighs if need be. Bring them up to shoulder height and hold them horizontally. Push both dumbbells up into the air and gently touch them together at the top of the movement. Slowly bring them back down to shoulder height and repeat this movement for the full sets and reps.

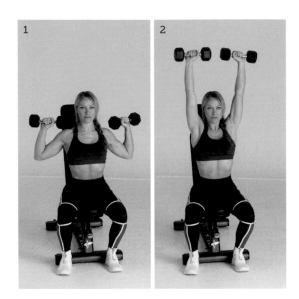

E 3 sets » 15 reps » 1 minute rest between sets

H 4 sets » 12 reps » 1 minute rest between sets

S 5 sets » 5 reps » 3 minute rest between sets

Lateral Raises
Heavy dumbbells

Make sure the weight is the same in each hand. Stand up straight with your knees slightly bent and your feet together. Grip the dumbbells in front of your crotch, lightly touching each other. Lean ever-so-slightly forward with your upper body, keeping a slight arch in your lower back. Keeping a slight bend in your elbows and bowing them outwards slightly, slowly and gradually raise the dumbbells out either side of you, until your arms are horizontal, like an eagle in flight. Hold this position for a fraction of a second, then slowly bring your arms back down to your starting position. Take a breath and repeat this movement for the full amount of sets and reps.

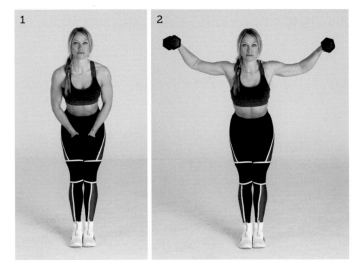

E 3 sets » 15 reps » 1 minute rest between sets

H 4 sets » 12 reps » 1 minute rest between sets

Front Raises Heavy dumbbells

Make sure the weight is the same in each hand. Stand up straight with your feet hip-width apart and your toes pointing forwards. Grip the dumbbells horizontally, using an overhand grip, and allow them to hang together in front of your crotch. Keeping your back straight at all times, take a deep breath and slowly raise one of the dumbbells. Keep a slight bend in your elbow as you do so. Hold the dumbbell in its raised position for a fraction of a second, then slowly bring it back down. Repeat with the other arm. Continue this movement alternately for the full amount of sets and reps.

E 3 sets » 15 reps » 1 minute rest between sets

H 4 sets » 12 reps » 1 minute rest between sets

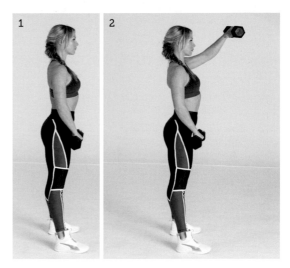

Bent Over Rows with Olympic Bar Heavy weight

Stand up straight with your feet hip-width apart. Grab the bar with both hands and pull your shoulders back. Keeping an arch in your back and holding the bar against your lower body, slowly come down into a hamstring stretch until you have reached your full range of motion. Once there, pull the bar up into your ribcage, then slowly lower it back down again. Take a deep breath and repeat this movement for the full amount of sets and reps.

E 3 sets » 15 reps » 1 minute rest between sets

H 4 sets » 12 reps » 1 minute rest between sets

S 5 sets » 5 reps » 3 minutes rest between sets

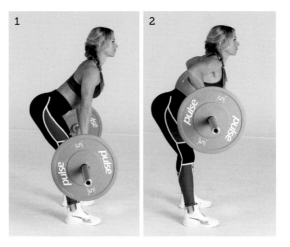

Bicep Curls Heavy dumbbells

Stand up straight with your feet hip-width apart. Grip a dumbbell in each hand and allow them to hang either side of your hips. Keeping your arms in tight to your sides at all times, slowly lift the dumbbells from hip height into your shoulders, twisting the dumbbells into a horizontal position as you do so. Slowly lower the dumbbells back down to their starting position. Continue this movement for the full amount of sets and reps.

E 3 sets » 15 reps » 1 minute rest between sets

H 4 sets » 12 reps » 1 minute rest between sets

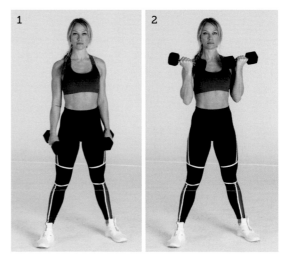

Tuesday + Friday Upper Body

Chest Press with Olympic Bar
Heavy weight

(I would rather you use a bench press – a bench underneath a racked Olympic bar – for chest press exercies. However, if you have to use a Smith machine – illustrated here – that's fine.) Make sure the weight is the same each side of the bar – use clips if you need to. Lie back on the bench with your feet either side and flat on the floor. Reaching up, grip the bar with both hands – your hands should be directly above your shoulders. Push the bar up so it is free from the holding, then bring it down slowly so it lightly touches your chest. Push the bar back up into the air and hold it there for a second before bringing it back down. Repeat this movement for the full amount of sets and reps.

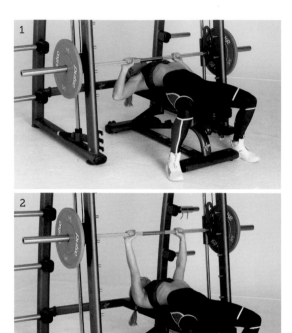

E 3 sets » 15 reps » 1 minute rest between sets

H 4 sets » 12 reps » 1 minute rest between sets

S 5 sets » 5 reps » 3 minute rest between sets

Tricep Dips on Machine Assisted

Make sure the padded seat is upright and the bars on either side of the machine are as close together as possible (they are often adjustable). Facing the machine, grip the bars and place your knees on top of the padded seat. Keeping your elbows in tight to your sides, slowly allow your body to drop down. When you have come down as far as possible, slowly push yourself back up, using your triceps. Take a deep breath and repeat this movement for the full amount of sets and reps.

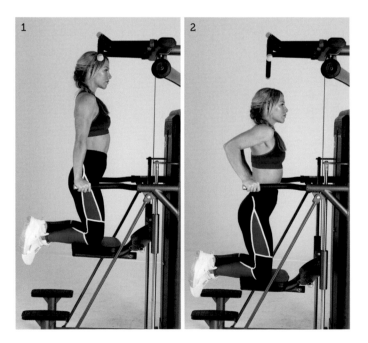

E 3 sets » 15 reps »
1 minute rest between sets

H 4 sets » 12 reps »
1 minute rest between sets

Wednesday + Saturday Back/Core

Hyperextensions on Machine
Heavy weight

(Please note that the illustration shows an unweighted hyperextension on the mat. If your gym has a hyperextension machine, though, this is preferable. Hold a weight plate against your chest as you do the hyperextensions on the machine.) Slowly bow your body back into a lower back crunch (another name for this exercise is a reverse sit up). Make sure you engage your glutes and core while doing this exercise. Hold this position for a few seconds then repeat this movement for the full amount of sets and reps.

E 3 sets » 15 reps » 1 minute rest between sets

H 4 sets » 12 reps » 1 minute rest between sets

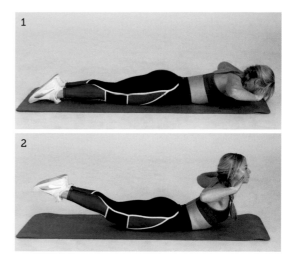

Dumbbell Pullovers on Bench
Heavy dumbbell

Sit on the bench, legs either side of it, and grip the dumbbell (vertically) between your legs. Lie down and, as you do so, raise the dumbbell up in the air, directly above your face. Now adjust your grip by opening your hands, allowing the weight of the dumbbell to rest against the flats of your palms, gripping around its base with your fingers. Allow the dumbbell to slowly and gently come behind you, so that it is behind your head and behind the bench. Slowly and gently bring it back up into the air, above your face, into your starting position. Take a deep breath and repeat this movement for the full amount of sets and reps.

E 3 sets » 15 reps » 1 minute rest between sets

H 4 sets » 12 reps » 1 minute rest between sets

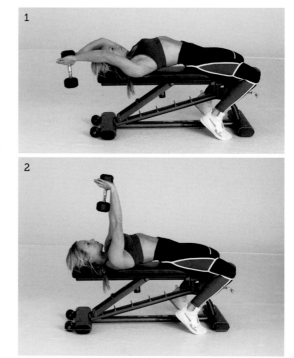

Wednesday + Saturday Back/Core

Wide Grip Rows on Machine Heavy weight

You can do these on a static machine or using the cable machine (as illustrated), depending on what equipment your gym has. Either sit with your legs either side of the machine or stand with your feet together and knees bent. Holding the bar using an overhand grip, take a deep breath and slowly and gently pull the bar into your chest. Hold it against yourself for a second, then slowly and gently let it pull you back to the starting position. Take a deep breath and repeat this movement for the full amount of sets and reps.

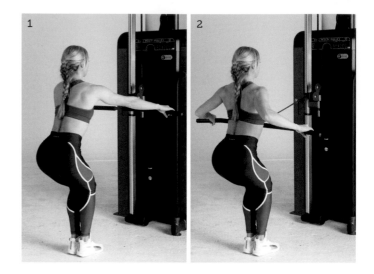

E 3 sets » 15 reps »
1 minute rest between sets

H 4 sets » 12 reps »
1 minute rest between sets

Close Grip Rows on Machine Heavy weight

You can do these on a static machine (as illustrated) or using the cable machine, depending on what equipment your gym has. Sit down with your legs either side of the machine and grip the handles in front of you with an inverted grip. Take a deep breath and, slowly and gently, pull the handles into your chest. Hold the handles against yourself for a second, then slowly and gently let them pull you back to the starting position. Take a deep breath and repeat this movement for the full amount of sets and reps.

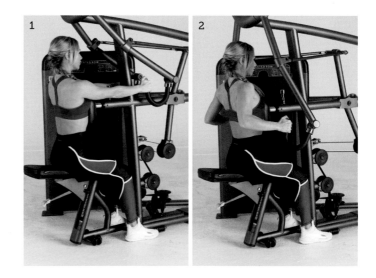

E 3 sets » 15 reps »
1 minute rest between sets

H 4 sets » 12 reps »
1 minute rest between sets

Wide Grip Pullups on Machine Fully assisted

Make sure the padded seat is upright. Facing the machine, grip the bars that are furthest apart using an overhand grip and place your knees on top of the padded seat. Slowly allow your body to drop down underneath the bars. Once your arms are fully extended, slowly pull yourself back up into a wide-grip pull-up position. Hold this for a second before allowing yourself to come back down to your starting position. Take a deep breath and repeat this movement for the full amount of sets and reps.

E 3 sets » 15 reps »
1 minute rest between sets

H 4 sets » 12 reps »
1 minute rest between sets

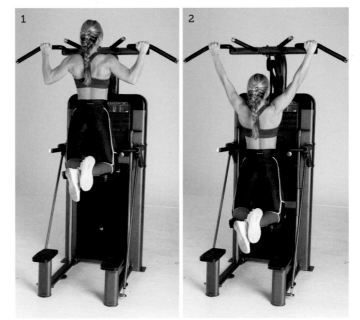

Close Grip Pullups on Machine Fully assisted

Make sure the padded seat is upright. Facing the machine, grip the bars above you that are closest together using an underhand grip. Place your knees on top of the padded seat, then slowly allow your body to drop down underneath the bars. Once your arms are fully extended, slowly pull yourself back up into a pull-up position. Hold this position for a second before allowing yourself to come back down again. Take a deep breath and repeat this movement for the full amount of sets and reps.

E 3 sets » 15 reps »
1 minute rest between sets

H 4 sets » 12 reps »
1 minute rest between sets

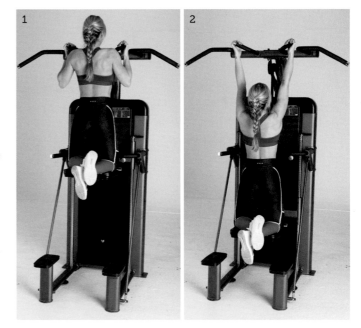

SUNDAY = FULL REST DAY

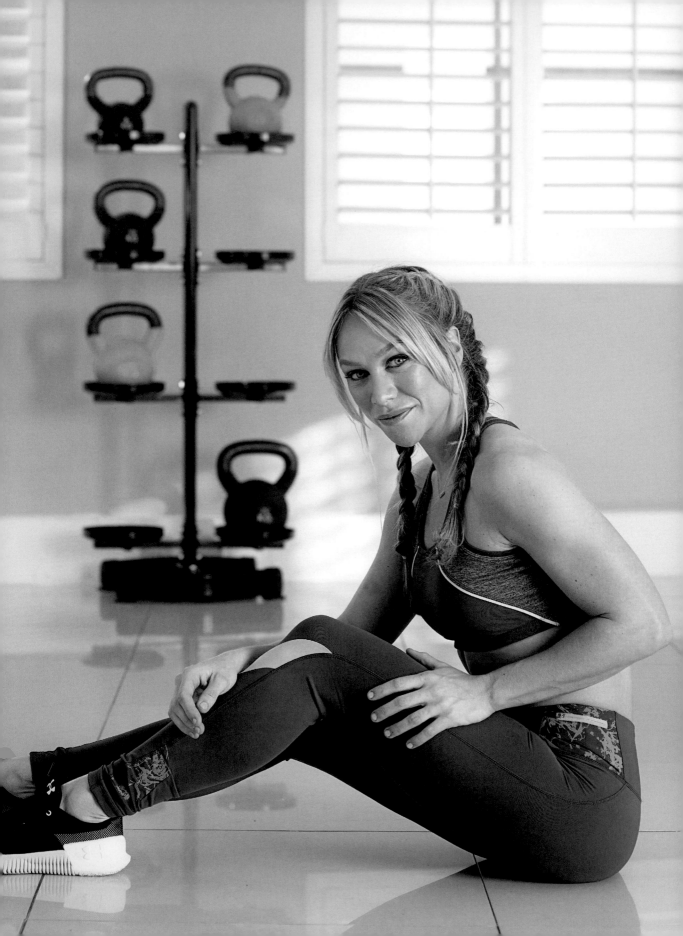

INTERMEDIATE

If you have lifted weights for a while but deep down you know your form isn't great, then I want you to start with the Beginner Plan. Go back to basics, train like you really are a newbie and learn the right form before making your way to the Intermediate Plan. That said, if you can lift and you know your form is great then this is the section for you!

The Intermediate Plan starts relatively simply and progresses slowly over the 4 weeks.

You will already know that every good weight-lifting plan includes four staple lifts:

- Squats
- Rows
- Deadlifts
- Presses

These big, compound, push/pull movements are going to hit your body in multiple ways that other, more isolated, exercises will not. There is a time and a place for more isolated work, and you will see that in this plan, too.

Please note – no one can tell you what weight to lift other than your own body. I want you to start at a weight you know you can handle before you even think about increasing it.

Always remember that form is *primary* and weight is *secondary*.

Choosing Your Weight-training Goal

Endurance Training *(the muscle's ability to generate force repeatedly)* is perfect for those wanting to increase their 'functional' training abilities, such as triathletes, distance runners and rowers. If you are a cardio bunny looking to implement some weight lifting to assist your sport, then endurance is perfect for you.

Hypertrophy Training *(the growth of a muscle)* is perfect for those wanting to increase visible muscle mass, and is my favourite form of weight lifting. If you are looking for aesthetic muscular results, hypertrophy is for you.

Strength Training *(the muscle's ability to generate force against resistance)* or powerlifting is perfect for those wanting to increase their physical strength and really enjoy their weight lifting. It traditionally only calls for 3 exercises – squat, deadlift and bench press, as these are the competition lifts. However, in recent years 2 common exercises have been included in the training – military press and barbell row.

I have written the exercise plans to cover all the bases so there are 2 days for each different area of the body (upper, lower and back / core). As a result, each plan has 6 days a week of training BUT you do not need to train for the full 6 days. As long as you train your body evenly (don't just focus on legs, for example), feel free to weight-train anywhere between 4 and 6 times a week, taking rest days as and when you need them. This advice is especially important with strength training – recovery is key for this goal, so training 4 days a week is enough.

Try not to train the same body part 2 days in a row, as you want to give each muscle group at least 24 hours to recover after training.

When I instruct a *Comfortable Weight*, I mean a weight that challenges you but that you can lift with ease.

When I instruct a *Heavy Weight*, I mean a weight that challenges you to really push HARD by your last few reps.

You can repeat this plan for as many weeks / months as you wish. However, at some point, it would be good to progress to the Advanced Plan...

Week 1 Getting Comfortable
(form with weight focused)

Monday + Thursday = Lower Body

Tuesday + Friday = Upper Body

Wednesday + Saturday = Back/Core

Sunday = Rest day

You'll see this is a 6-day weight-lifting plan. However, you only need to train for 4 or 5 days a week, if you'd prefer.

As long as you make sure you train your body evenly – at least 1 day on your Lower Body, 1 day on your Upper Body and 1 day on your Back/Core – feel free to weight-train anywhere between 4 and 6 days a week, taking rest days as and when you need them.

Key to symbols

E Endurance

H Hypertrophy

 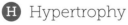

S Strength. If Strength is your goal but the symbol is missing from an exercise, leave the exercise out.

Monday + Thursday Lower Body

Squats on Smith Machine Comfortable weight

(Please note: the illustration shows the Smith unweighted – this exercise should be weighted.) Make sure the weight is the same on each side. Find the centre of the horizontal bar and duck underneath it, so the bar is resting across your shoulders. Place your feet hip-width apart, or slightly further if that is more comfortable, and make sure your toes are either pointing forwards or slightly outwards. Take hold of the bar either side of your shoulders and unhook it from the machine – keep it unhooked using your grip. Standing up straight and bending only at the hips and knees, come down into a low squat before pushing back up through your heels to a standing position, squeezing your glutes as you do so. Take a breath and repeat this movement for the full amount of sets and reps.

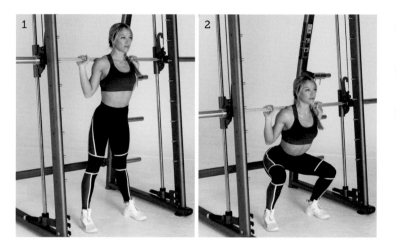

E 3 sets » 15 reps »
1 minute rest between sets

H 4 sets » 12 reps »
1 minute rest between sets

S 5 sets » 5 reps »
1 minute rest between sets

Bulgarian Split Squats on Smith Machine Comfortable weight

(Please note: the illustration shows the Smith unweighted – this exercise should be weighted.) Place the bench about 0.5m behind you. Find the centre of the horizontal bar and duck underneath it, so the bar is resting across your shoulders. Place one foot up on the bench behind you, resting top down. Make sure the toes of your standing foot are pointing forwards. Take hold of the bar either side of your shoulders and unhook the bar from the machine – keep it unhooked using your grip. Standing up straight and bending only at the hip and knee, come down into a low squat before pushing back up through your heel to a standing position. Take a breath and repeat on the other leg. Repeat for the full amount of sets and reps.

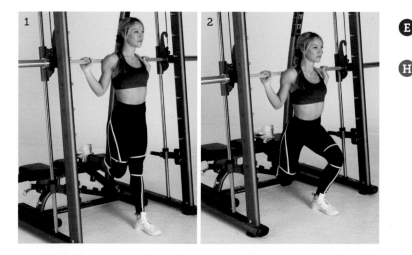

E 3 sets » 15 reps »
1 minute rest between sets

H 4 sets » 12 reps »
1 minute rest between sets

Monday + Thursday Lower Body

Hip Thrusts on Smith Machine Comfortable weight

(Please note: the illustration shows the Smith unweighted – this exercise should be weighted.)
Place the bench about 0.5m behind you, so you are sandwiched between the Smith and the bench.
Lower the bar so it is about 30cm off the ground. Sit down on the floor between the bar and the bench,
facing the bar and resting your upper back and shoulder blades on the edge of the bench. Place a bar
pad (a black, cushioned tube) around the centre of the horizontal bar. Place your feet hip-width apart
and keep your toes pointing forwards or slightly outwards. Place your hips underneath the cushion and
your hands either side of your hips. Unhook the bar from the machine – keep it unhooked using your
grip – and thrust up into the air, through your glutes, squeezing them tight at the top of the movement.
Hold this position for a few seconds before coming back down until your buttocks are just above the
ground. Take a breath and repeat this movement for the full amount of sets and reps.

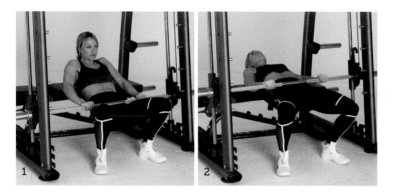

E 3 sets **»** 15 reps **»**
1 minute rest between sets

H 4 sets **»** 12 reps **»**
1 minute rest between sets

Deadlift with Olympic Bar
Comfortable weight

Make sure the weight is the same each side – use
clips if you need to. Place the bar in front of your
feet. Stand up straight with your feet hip-width
apart, toes pointing forwards. Keeping your back
straight and bending only at the hips and knees,
crouch down so your hands are able to reach the
bar. Grasp the bar either side of your legs, placing
one hand in an overhand grip and the other in an
underhand grip (whichever is more comfortable
is fine). Once you have a good grip, stand up
straight, pushing down through your heels as
you do so. As you come into a fully vertical
standing position, squeeze your buttocks at the
top of the movement. Keeping the bar against
your legs, slowly allow it to pull you back down
to the ground again, keeping your back straight
and bending only at the hips and knees at all times.
Allow the bar to hit the floor, take a breath and
repeat the lift for the full amount of sets and reps.

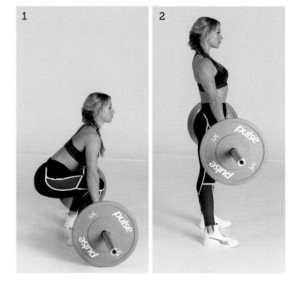

E 3 sets **»** 15 reps **»** 1 minute rest between sets

H 4 sets **»** 12 reps **»** 1 minute rest between sets

S 5 sets **»** 5 reps **»** 1 minute rest between sets

Romanian Deadlift with Olympic Bar Comfortable weight

Make sure the weight is the same each side – use clips if you need to. Place the bar in front of your feet. Stand up straight with your feet hip-width apart and your toes pointing forwards. Keeping your back straight and bending only at the hips and knees, crouch down to grasp the bar. Grasp it either side of your legs, placing one hand in an overhand grip, the other in an underhand grip (whichever hand is more comfortable). Stand up straight, pushing down through your heels as you do so. As you come into a full standing position, squeeze your buttocks at the top of the movement. Pull your shoulders back and keep them back during the exercise. Engage your core and make sure to keep your entire core and back position solid throughout. Keeping the bar against your legs, slowly allow it to pull you down from the hips as far as your hamstrings will allow – sticking your bottom out as you go. Take a breath and return to your starting position. Repeat the lift for the full amount of sets and reps.

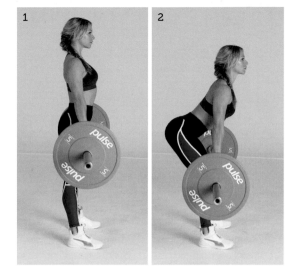

E 3 sets » 15 reps » 1 minute rest between sets

H 4 sets » 12 reps » 1 minute rest between sets

Leg Press on Machine
Comfortable weight

Sit down and place your feet hip-width apart on the plate in front of you (or slightly further apart if that is more comfortable). Point your toes upwards, or slightly outwards. Pushing through the flats of your feet, slowly and gently push against the plate. Depending on the machine, the force will either push the plate away from your seat, or your seat away from the plate. When you have fully extended (without locking your knees out – you should always keep a slight bend in them when performing a lower body lift), slowly come back into your starting position. Take a breath and repeat this movement for the full amount of sets and reps. Finish with light calf presses to exhaust. (Lower your feet to the bottom of the plate and push on to the balls of your feet. Flex your foot so your heels come back down again, then repeat to exhaust.)

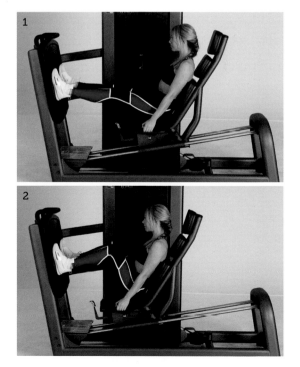

E 3 sets » 15 reps » 1 minute rest between sets

H 4 sets » 12 reps » 1 minute rest between sets

Tuesday + Friday Upper Body

Seated Dumbbell Press
Comfortable dumbbells

Adjust the bench so it's upright then sit up straight on the bench with your back against it. Hold a dumbbell in each hand and rest them on top of your thighs if need be. Bring them up to shoulder height and hold them horizontally. Push both dumbbells up into the air and gently touch them together at the top of the movement. Slowly bring them back down to shoulder height and repeat this movement for the full sets and reps.

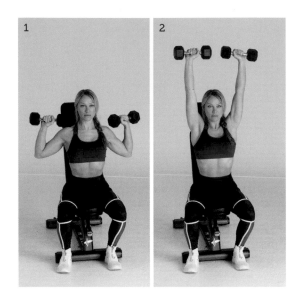

E 3 sets » 15 reps » 1 minute rest between sets

H 4 sets » 12 reps » 1 minute rest between sets

S 5 sets » 5 reps » 1 minute rest between sets

Lateral Raises
Comfortable dumbbells

Make sure the weight is the same in each hand. Stand up straight with your knees slightly bent and your feet together. Grip the dumbbells in front of your crotch, lightly touching each other. Lean ever-so-slightly forward with your upper body, keeping a slight arch in your lower back. Keeping a slight bend in your elbows and bowing them outwards slightly, slowly and gradually raise the dumbbells out either side of you, until your arms are horizontal, like an eagle in flight. Hold this position for a fraction of a second, then slowly bring your arms back down to your starting position. Take a breath and repeat this movement for the full amount of sets and reps.

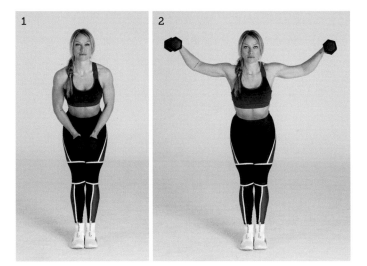

E 3 sets » 15 reps » 1 minute rest between sets

H 4 sets » 12 reps » 1 minute rest between sets

Front Raises
Comfortable dumbbells

Make sure the weight is the same in each hand. Stand up straight with your feet hip-width apart and your toes pointing forwards. Grip the dumbbells horizontally, using an overhand grip, and allow them to hang together in front of your crotch. Keeping your back straight at all times, take a deep breath and slowly raise one of the dumbbells. Keep a slight bend in your elbow as you do so. Hold the dumbbell in its raised position for a fraction of a second, then slowly bring it back down. Repeat with the other arm. Continue this movement alternately for the full amount of sets and reps.

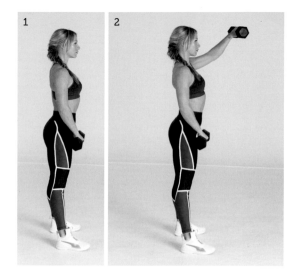

(E) 3 sets **»** 15 reps **»** 1 minute rest between sets

(H) 4 sets **»** 12 reps **»** 1 minute rest between sets

Bent Over Rows with
Dumbbell Comfortable dumbbell

Place a dumbbell on the floor on the right-hand side of a bench. Keeping your right foot on the ground and your toes pointing forwards, place your left knee in the centre of the bench, then bend over and grip the top of the bench with your left hand. Keeping your back straight, slowly pick up the dumbbell with your right hand, making sure to keep your arm in tight to your body as you do so. Pull the dumbbell up into your armpit region and hold the dumbbell there for a fraction of a second, then slowly bring it back down to extend your arm. Continue this movement for the full amount of sets and reps, then repeat with the other arm.

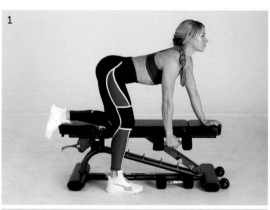

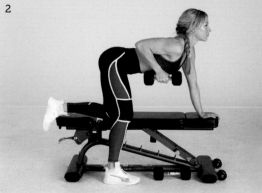

(E) 3 sets **»** 15 reps **»** 1 minute rest between sets

(H) 4 sets **»** 12 reps **»** 1 minute rest between sets

(S) 5 sets **»** 5 reps **»** 1 minute rest between sets

Tuesday + Friday Upper Body

Chest Press with Olympic Bar
Comfortable weight

(I would rather you use a bench press – a bench underneath a racked Olympic bar – for chest press exercies. However, if you have to use a Smith machine – illustrated here – that's fine.) Make sure the weight is the same each side of the bar – use clips if you need to. Lie back on the bench with your feet either side and flat against the floor. Reaching up, grip the bar with both your hands – your hands should be directly above your shoulders. Push the bar up so it is free from the holding, then bring it down slowly so it lightly touches your chest. Push the bar back up into the air and hold it there for a second before bringing it back down. Repeat this exercise for the full amount of sets and reps.

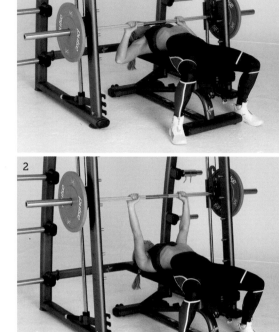

(E) 3 sets » 15 reps » 1 minute rest between sets

(H) 4 sets » 12 reps » 1 minute rest between sets

(S) 5 sets » 5 reps » 1 minute rest between sets

Chest Fly on Bench
Comfortable dumbbells

Make sure the weight is the same in each hand. Sit on the bench with your feet flat on the floor on either side and grip the dumbbells in your hands, resting them on top of your thighs. Lie down on the bench. Extend your arms out either side of your body at chest height. Then, as if you are hugging a beach ball, and keeping a slight bend in your elbows, bring the dumbbells together above your body. Slowly bring the dumbbells back down to the starting position. Take a breath and repeat this movement for the full amount of sets and reps.

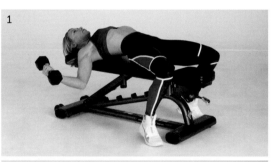

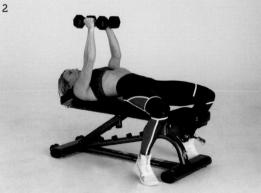

(E) 3 sets » 15 reps » 1 minute rest between sets

(H) 4 sets » 12 reps » 1 minute rest between sets

Wednesday + Saturday Back/Core

Hyperextensions on Machine
Comfortable weight

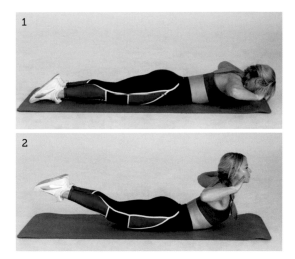

(Please note that the illustration shows an unweighted hyperextension on the mat. If your gym has a hyperextension machine, though, this is preferable. Hold a weight plate against your chest as you do the hyperextensions on the machine.) Slowly bow your body back into a lower back crunch (another name for this exercise is a reverse sit up). Make sure you engage your glutes and core while doing this exercise. Hold this position for a few seconds then repeat this movement for the full amount of sets and reps.

(**E**) 3 sets » 15 reps » 1 minute rest between sets

(**H**) 4 sets » 12 reps » 1 minute rest between sets

Dumbbell Pullovers on Bench
Comfortable dumbbell

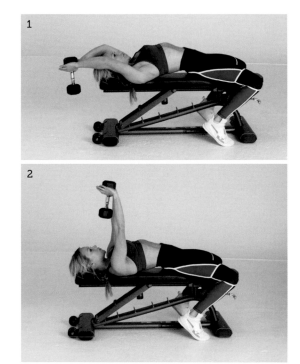

Sit on the bench, legs either side of it, and grip the dumbbell (vertically) between your legs. Lie down and, as you do so, raise the dumbbell up in the air, directly above your face. Now adjust your grip by opening your hands, allowing the weight of the dumbbell to rest against the flats of your palms, gripping around its base with your fingers. Allow the dumbbell to slowly and gently come behind you, so that it is behind your head and behind the bench. Slowly and gently bring it back up into the air, above your face, into your starting position. Take a deep breath and repeat this movement for the full amount of sets and reps.

(**E**) 3 sets » 15 reps » 1 minute rest between sets

(**H**) 4 sets » 12 reps » 1 minute rest between sets

Wednesday + Saturday Back/Core

Wide Grip Rows on Machine Comfortable weight

You can do these on a static machine or using the cable machine (as illustrated), depending on what equipment your gym has. Either sit with your legs either side of the machine or stand with your feet together and knees bent. Holding the bar using an overhand grip, take a deep breath and slowly and gently pull the bar into your chest. Hold it against yourself for a second, then slowly and gently let it pull you back to the starting position. Take a deep breath and repeat this movement for the full amount of sets and reps.

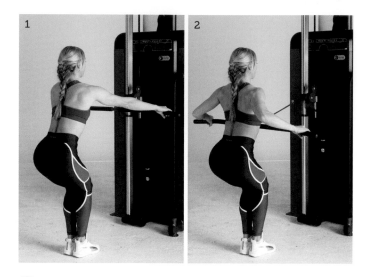

E 3 sets » 15 reps » 1 minute rest between sets

H 4 sets » 12 reps » 1 minute rest between sets

Close Grip Rows on Machine Comfortable weight

You can do these on a static machine (as illustrated) or using the cable machine, depending on what equipment your gym has. Sit down with your legs either side of the machine and grip the handles in front of you with an inverted grip. Take a deep breath and, slowly and gently, pull the handles into your chest. Hold the handles against yourself for a second, then slowly and gently let them pull you back to the starting position. Take a deep breath and repeat this movement for the full amount of sets and reps.

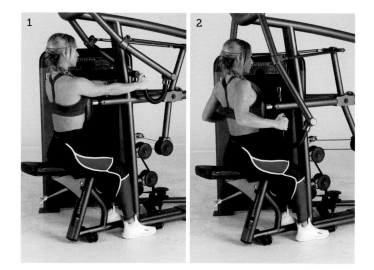

E 3 sets » 15 reps » 1 minute rest between sets

H 4 sets » 12 reps » 1 minute rest between sets

Wide Grip Pullups on Machine Assisted

Make sure the padded seat is upright. Facing the machine, grip the bars that are furthest apart using an overhand grip and place your knees on top of the padded seat. Slowly allow your body to drop down underneath the bars. Once your arms are fully extended, slowly pull yourself back up into a wide-grip pull-up position. Hold this for a second before allowing yourself to come back down to your starting position. Take a deep breath and repeat this movement for the full amount of sets and reps.

E 3 sets » 15 reps »
1 minute rest between sets

H 4 sets » 12 reps »
1 minute rest between sets

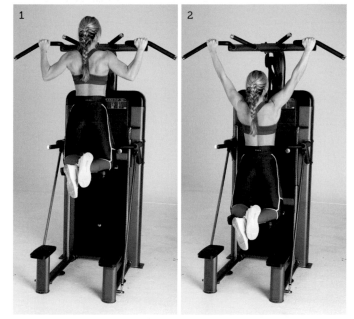

Close Grip Pullups on Machine Assisted

Make sure the padded seat is upright. Facing the machine, grip the bars above you that are closest together using an underhand grip. Place your knees on top of the padded seat, then slowly allow your body to drop down underneath the bars. Once your arms are fully extended, slowly pull yourself back up into a pull-up position. Hold this position for a second before allowing yourself to come back down again. Take a deep breath and repeat this movement for the full amount of sets and reps.

E 3 sets » 15 reps »
1 minute rest between sets

H 4 sets » 12 reps »
1 minute rest between sets

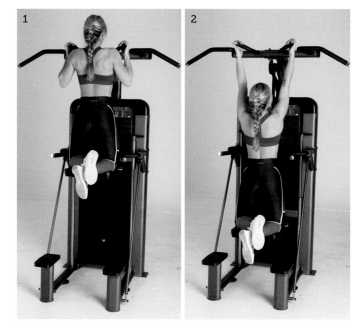

SUNDAY = FULL REST DAY

Week 2 Progressing
(comfortable and heavy weight focused)

Monday + Thursday = Lower Body

Tuesday + Friday = Upper Body

Wednesday + Saturday = Back/Core

Sunday = Rest day

You'll see this is a 6-day weight-lifting plan. However, you only need to train for 4 or 5 days a week, if you'd prefer.

As long as you make sure you train your body evenly – at least 1 day on your Lower Body, 1 day on your Upper Body and 1 day on your Back/Core – feel free to weight-train anywhere between 4 and 6 days a week, taking rest days as and when you need them.

Key to symbols

E Endurance

H Hypertrophy

S Strength. If Strength is your goal but the symbol is missing from an exercise, leave the exercise out.

Monday + Thursday Lower Body

Squats on Squat Rack with Olympic Bar Comfortable weight

Make sure the weight is the same on either side of the bar – use clips if you need to. Find the centre of the horizontal bar and duck underneath it, so the bar is resting across your shoulders. Take hold of the bar either side of your shoulders and come up slightly on your tiptoes. Remove the bar from its holdings and take a few cautious steps backwards. Place your feet hip-width apart, or slightly further if that is a more comfortable squat position for you, and make sure your toes are either pointing forwards or slightly outwards, whichever is more comfortable. Standing up straight and bending only at the hip and knees, come down into a low squat before pushing back up through your heels to a standing position, squeezing your glutes as you do so. Take a breath and repeat this movement for the full amount of sets and reps.

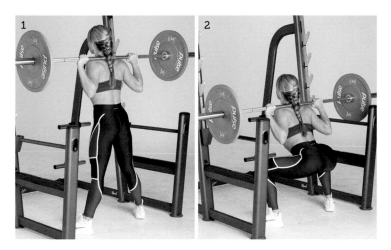

E 3 sets » 15 reps »
1 minute rest between sets

H 4 sets » 12 reps »
1 minute rest between sets

S 5 sets » 5 reps »
1 minute rest between sets

Bulgarian Split Squats on Smith Machine Heavy weight

(Please note: the illustration shows the Smith unweighted – this exercise should be weighted.) Place the bench about 0.5m behind you. Find the centre of the horizontal bar and duck underneath it, so the bar is resting across your shoulders. Place one foot up on the bench behind you, resting top down. Make sure the toes of your standing foot are pointing forwards. Take hold of the bar either side of your shoulders and unhook the bar from the machine – keep it unhooked using your grip. Standing up straight and bending only at the hip and knee, come down into a low squat before pushing back up through your heel to a standing position. Take a breath and repeat on the other leg. Repeat for the full amount of sets and reps.

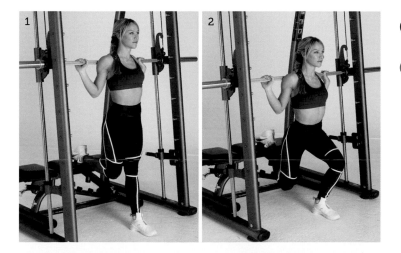

E 3 sets » 15 reps »
1 minute rest between sets

H 4 sets » 12 reps »
1 minute rest between sets

Monday + Thursday Lower Body

Hip Thrusts on Smith Machine Heavy weight

(Please note: the illustration shows the Smith unweighted – this exercise should be weighted.) Place the bench about 0.5m behind you, so you are sandwiched between the Smith and the bench. Lower the bar so it is about 30cm off the ground. Sit down on the floor between the bar and the bench, facing the bar and resting your upper back and shoulder blades on the edge of the bench. Place a bar pad (a black, cushioned tube) around the centre of the horizontal bar. Place your feet hip-width apart and keep your toes pointing forwards or slightly outwards. Place your hips underneath the cushion and your hands either side of your hips. Unhook the bar from the machine – keep it unhooked using your grip – and thrust up into the air, through your glutes, squeezing them tight at the top of the movement. Hold this position for a few seconds before coming back down until your buttocks are just above the ground. Take a breath and repeat this movement for the full amount of sets and reps.

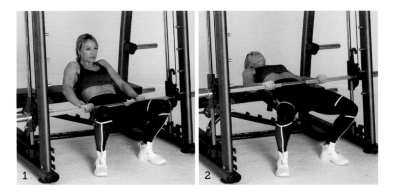

E 3 sets » 15 reps »
1 minute rest between sets

H 4 sets » 12 reps »
1 minute rest between sets

Deadlift with Olympic Bar
Heavy weight

Make sure the weight is the same each side – use clips if you need to. Place the bar in front of your feet. Stand up straight with your feet hip-width apart, toes pointing forwards. Keeping your back straight and bending only at the hips and knees, crouch down so your hands are able to reach the bar. Grasp the bar either side of your legs, placing one hand in an overhand grip and the other in an underhand grip (whichever is more comfortable is fine). Once you have a good grip, stand up straight, pushing down through your heels as you do so. As you come into a fully vertical standing position, squeeze your buttocks at the top of the movement. Keeping the bar against your legs, slowly allow it to pull you back down to the ground again, keeping your back straight and bending only at the hips and knees at all times. Allow the bar to hit the floor, take a breath and repeat the lift for the full amount of sets and reps.

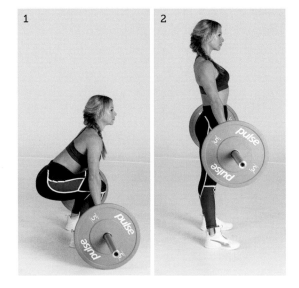

E 3 sets » 15 reps » 1 minute rest between sets

H 4 sets » 12 reps » 1 minute rest between sets

S 5 sets » 5 reps » 3 minutes rest between sets

Romanian Deadlift with Olympic Bar Heavy weight

Make sure the weight is the same each side – use clips if you need to. Place the bar in front of your feet. Stand up straight with your feet hip-width apart and your toes pointing forwards. Keeping your back straight and bending only at the hips and knees, crouch down so your hands are now able to grasp the bar. Grasp it either side of your legs, placing one hand in an overhand grip, the other in an underhand grip (whichever hand is more comfortable is fine). Once you have a good grip on the bar, stand up straight, pushing down through your heels as you do so. As you come into a full standing position, squeeze your buttocks at the top of the movement. Pull your shoulders back and keep them back during this exercise. Engage your core and make sure to keep your entire core and back position solid throughout. Keeping the bar against your legs, slowly allow it to pull you down from the hips as far as your hamstrings will allow – sticking your bottom out as you go. Take a breath and return to your starting position. Repeat the lift for the full amount of sets and reps.

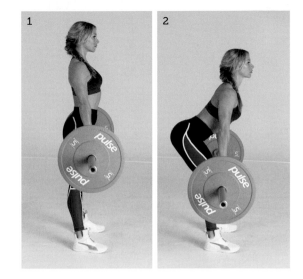

E 3 sets » 15 reps » 1 minute rest between sets

H 4 sets » 12 reps » 1 minute rest between sets

Leg Press on Machine
Heavy weight

Sit down and place your feet hip-width apart on the plate in front of you (or slightly further apart if that is more comfortable). Point your toes upwards, or slightly outwards. Pushing through the flats of your feet, slowly and gently push against the plate. Depending on the machine, the force will either push the plate away from your seat, or your seat away from the plate. When you have fully extended (without locking your knees out – you should always keep a slight bend in them when performing a lower body lift), slowly come back into your starting position. Take a breath and repeat this movement for the full amount of sets and reps. Finish with light calf presses to exhaust.

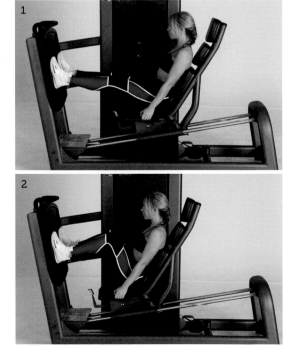

E 3 sets » 15 reps » 1 minute rest between sets

H 4 sets » 12 reps » 1 minute rest between sets

Tuesday + Friday Upper Body

Seated Dumbbell Press
Heavy dumbbells

Adjust the bench so it's upright then sit up straight on the bench with your back against it. Hold a dumbbell in each hand and rest them on top of your thighs if need be. Bring them up to shoulder height and hold them horizontally. Push both dumbbells up into the air and gently touch them together at the top of the movement. Slowly bring them back down to shoulder height and repeat this movement for the full sets and reps.

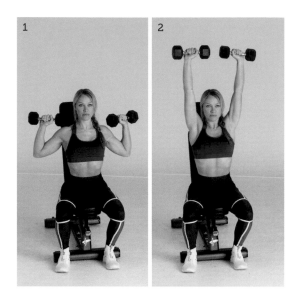

E 3 sets » 15 reps » 1 minute rest between sets

H 4 sets » 12 reps » 1 minute rest between sets

S 5 sets » 5 reps » 3 minutes rest between sets

Lateral Raises
Heavy dumbbells

Make sure the weight is the same in each hand. Stand up straight with your knees slightly bent and your feet together. Grip the dumbbells in front of your crotch, lightly touching each other. Lean ever-so-slightly forward with your upper body, keeping a slight arch in your lower back. Keeping a slight bend in your elbows and bowing them outwards slightly, slowly and gradually raise the dumbbells out either side of you, until your arms are horizontal, like an eagle in flight. Hold this position for a fraction of a second, then slowly bring your arms back down to your starting position. Take a breath and repeat this movement for the full amount of sets and reps.

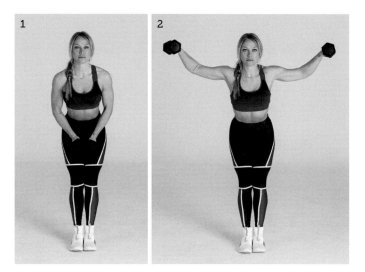

E 3 sets » 15 reps » 1 minute rest between sets

H 4 sets » 12 reps » 1 minute rest between sets

Front Raises Heavy dumbbells

Make sure the weight is the same in each hand. Stand up straight with your feet hip-width apart and your toes pointing forwards. Grip the dumbbells horizontally, using an overhand grip, and allow them to hang together in front of your crotch. Keeping your back straight at all times, take a deep breath and slowly raise one of the dumbbells. Keep a slight bend in your elbow as you do so. Hold the dumbbell in its raised position for a fraction of a second, then slowly bring it back down. Repeat with the other arm. Continue this movement alternately for the full amount of sets and reps.

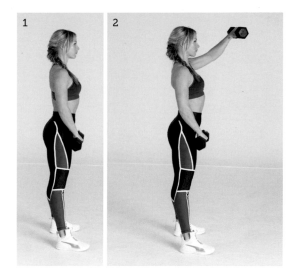

E 3 sets » 15 reps » 1 minute rest between sets

H 4 sets » 12 reps » 1 minute rest between sets

Bent Over Rows with Olympic Bar Heavy weight

Stand up straight with your feet hip-width apart. Grab the bar with both hands and pull your shoulders back. Keeping an arch in your back and holding the bar against your lower body, slowly come down into a hamstring stretch until you have reached your full range of motion. Once there, pull the bar up into your ribcage, then slowly lower it back down again. Take a deep breath and repeat this movement for the full amount of sets and reps.

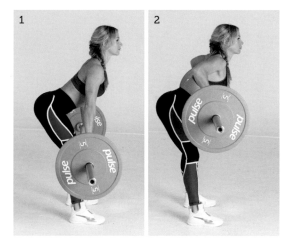

E 3 sets » 15 reps » 1 minute rest between sets

H 4 sets » 12 reps » 1 minute rest between sets

S 5 sets » 5 reps » 3 minutes rest between sets

Tuesday + Friday Upper Body

Chest Press with Olympic Bar Heavy weight

(I would rather you use a bench press – a bench underneath a racked Olympic bar – for chest press exercises. However, if you have to use a Smith machine – illustrated here – that's fine.) Make sure the weight is the same each side of the bar – use clips if you need to. Lie back on the bench with your feet either side and flat on the floor. Reaching up, grip the bar with both hands – your hands should be directly above your shoulders. Push the bar up so it is free from the holding, then bring it down slowly so it lightly touches your chest. Push the bar back up into the air and hold it there for a second before bringing it back down. Repeat this movement for the full amount of sets and reps.

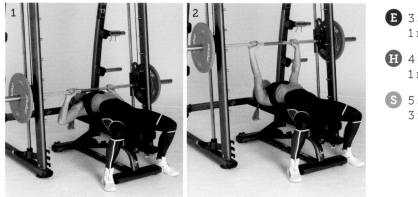

E 3 sets » 15 reps »
1 minute rest between sets

H 4 sets » 12 reps »
1 minute rest between sets

S 5 sets » 5 reps »
3 minutes rest between sets

Chest Fly on Bench
Heavy dumbbells

Make sure the weight is the same in each hand. Sit on the bench with your feet flat on the floor on either side and grip the dumbbells in your hands, resting them on top of your thighs. Lie down on the bench. Extend your arms out either side of your body at chest height. Then, as if you are hugging a beach ball, and keeping a slight bend in your elbows, bring the dumbbells together above your body. Slowly bring the dumbbells back down to the starting position. Take a breath and repeat this movement for the full amount of sets and reps.

E 3 sets » 15 reps » 1 minute rest between sets

H 4 sets » 12 reps » 1 minute rest between sets

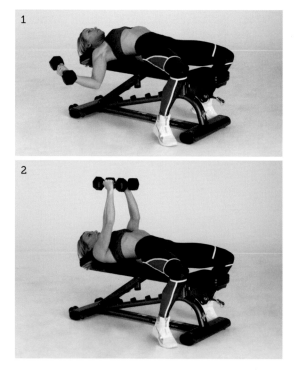

Wednesday + Saturday Back/Core

Hyperextensions on Machine
Heavy weight

(Please note that the illustration shows an unweighted hyperextension on the mat. If your gym has a hyperextension machine, though, this is preferable. Hold a weight plate against your chest as you do the hyperextensions on the machine.) Slowly bow your body back into a lower back crunch (another name for this exercise is a reverse sit up). Make sure you engage your glutes and core while doing this exercise. Hold this position for a few seconds then repeat this movement for the full amount of sets and reps.

E 3 sets » 15 reps » 1 minute rest between sets

H 4 sets » 12 reps » 1 minute rest between sets

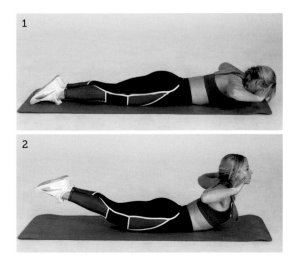

Dumbbell Pullovers on Bench
Heavy dumbbell

Sit on the bench, legs either side of it, and grip the dumbbell (vertically) between your legs. Lie down and, as you do so, raise the dumbbell up in the air, directly above your face. Now adjust your grip by opening your hands, allowing the weight of the dumbbell to rest against the flats of your palms, gripping around its base with your fingers. Allow the dumbbell to slowly and gently come behind you, so that it is both behind your head and behind the bench. Slowly and gently bring it back up into the air, above your face, into your starting position. Take a deep breath and repeat this movement for the full amount of sets and reps.

E 3 sets » 15 reps » 1 minute rest between sets

H 4 sets » 12 rep » 1 minute rest between sets

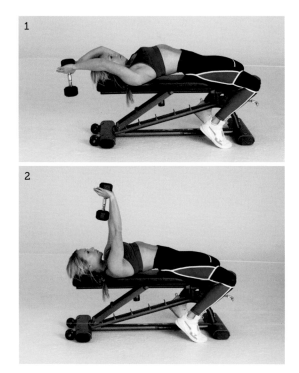

Wednesday + Saturday Back/Core

Wide Grip Rows on Machine Heavy weight

You can do these on a static machine or using the cable machine (as illustrated), depending on what equipment your gym has. Either sit with your legs either side of the machine or stand with your feet together and knees bent. Holding the bar using an overhand grip, take a deep breath and slowly and gently pull the bar into your chest. Hold it against yourself for a second, then slowly and gently let it pull you back to the starting position. Take a deep breath and repeat this movement for the full amount of sets and reps.

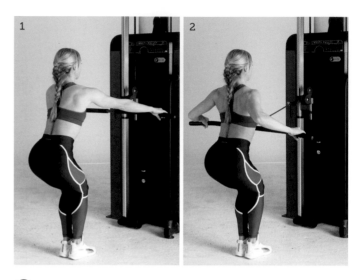

E 3 sets » 15 reps » 1 minute rest between sets

H 4 sets » 12 reps » 1 minute rest between sets

Close Grip Rows on Machine Heavy weight

You can do these on a static machine (as illustrated) or using the cable machine, depending on what equipment your gym has. Sit down with your legs either side of the machine and grip the handles in front of you with an inverted grip. Take a deep breath and, slowly and gently, pull the handles into your chest. Hold the handles against yourself for a second, then slowly and gently let them pull you back to the starting position. Take a deep breath and repeat this movement for the full amount of sets and reps.

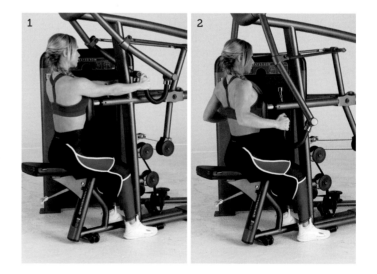

E 3 sets » 15 reps » 1 minute rest between sets

H 4 sets » 12 reps » 1 minute rest between sets

Wide Grip Pullups on Machine Assisted

Make sure the padded seat is upright. Facing the machine, grip the bars that are furthest apart using an overhand grip and place your knees on top of the padded seat. Slowly allow your body to drop down underneath the bars. Once your arms are fully extended, slowly pull yourself back up into a wide-grip pull-up position. Hold this for a second before allowing yourself to come back down to your starting position. Take a deep breath and repeat this movement for the full amount of sets and reps.

E 3 sets » 15 reps »
1 minute rest between sets

H 4 sets » 12 reps »
1 minute rest between sets

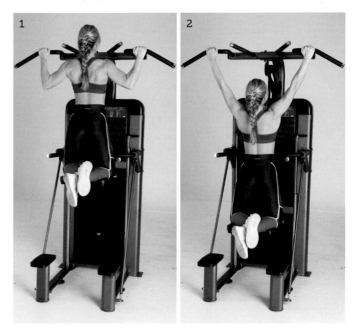

Close Grip Pullups on Machine Assisted

Make sure the padded seat is upright. Facing the machine, grip the bars above you that are closest together using an underhand grip. Place your knees on top of the padded seat, then slowly allow your body to drop down underneath the bars. Once your arms are fully extended, slowly pull yourself back up into a pull-up position. Hold this position for a second before allowing yourself to come back down again. Take a deep breath and repeat this movement for the full amount of sets and reps.

E 3 sets » 15 reps »
1 minute rest between sets

H 4 sets » 12 reps »
1 minute rest between sets

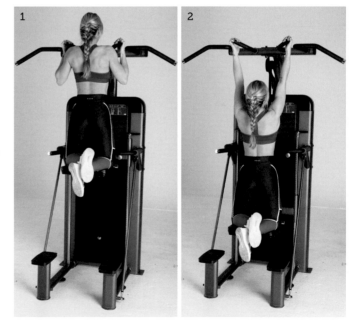

SUNDAY = FULL REST DAY

Intermediate

Week 3 Aim to Increase
(aim to increase weights if/when possible)

Monday + Thursday = Lower Body

Tuesday + Friday = Upper Body

Wednesday + Saturday = Back/Core

Sunday = Rest day

You'll see this is a 6-day weight-lifting plan. However, you only need to train for 4 or 5 days a week, if you'd prefer.

As long as you make sure you train your body evenly – at least 1 day on your Lower Body, 1 day on your Upper Body and 1 day on your Back/Core – feel free to weight-train anywhere between 4 and 6 days a week, taking rest days as and when you need them.

Key to symbols

E Endurance

H Hypertrophy

S Strength. If Strength is your goal but the symbol is missing from an exercise, leave the exercise out.

Monday + Thursday Lower Body

Squats on Squat Rack with Olympic Bar Heavy weight

Make sure the weight is the same on either side of the bar – use clips if you need to. Find the centre of the horizontal bar and duck underneath it, so the bar is resting across your shoulders. Take hold of the bar either side of your shoulders and come up slightly on your tiptoes. Remove the bar from its holdings and take a few cautious steps backwards. Place your feet hip-width apart, or slightly further if that is a more comfortable squat position for you, and make sure your toes are either pointing forwards or slightly outwards, whichever is more comfortable. Standing up straight and bending only at the hip and knees, come down into a low squat before pushing back up through your heels to a standing position, squeezing your glutes as you do so. Take a breath and repeat this movement for the full amount of sets and reps.

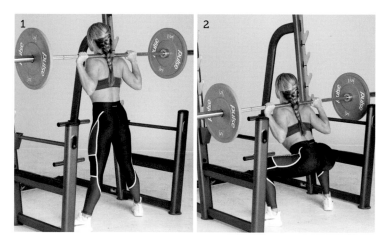

E 3 sets » 15 reps »
1 minute rest between sets

H 4 sets » 12 reps »
1 minute rest between sets

S 5 sets » 5 reps »
3 minutes rest between sets

Reverse Lunges on Smith Machine Heavy weight

(Please note: the illustration shows the Smith unweighted – this exercise should be weighted.) Make sure the weight is the same on each side of the bar. Find the centre of the horizontal bar and duck underneath it, so the bar is resting across your shoulders. Stand with your feet together. Place your hands on the bar either side of your shoulders and unhook the bar from the machine – keep it unhooked using your grip. Standing up straight, slowly step backwards with one of your feet, coming down into a low backwards lunge. As your back knee is just about to touch the ground, push back up and return to your starting position. Repeat immediately with the other leg. Continue this movement alternately for the full amount of sets and reps.

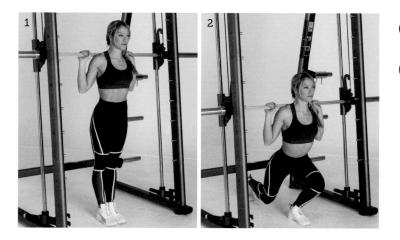

E 3 sets » 15 reps »
1 minute rest between sets

H 4 sets » 12 reps »
1 minute rest between sets

Monday + Thursday Lower Body

Glute Bridge Hold on Smith Machine Heavy weight

If you are new to lifting, you may not need to add a weight as this exercise is challenging unweighted. If you would like to try a weight, make sure it is the same on each side of the bar. Lower the bar down so it is about 30cm off the ground and place a bar pad (a black, cushioned tube) around the centre of the horizontal bar. Lie down underneath the bar with your hips directly under the bar pad. With your knees pointing upwards at a 90-degree angle, place your feet hip-width apart, or slightly further if that is more comfortable, and keep your toes pointing forwards or slightly outwards, whichever you prefer. Place your hips underneath the cushion and your hands either side of your hips, gripping the bar. Unhook the bar from the machine – keep it unhooked using your grip – and thrust up into the air, through your glutes, squeezing them tight at the top of the movement. Continue this movement for the full amount of sets and reps.

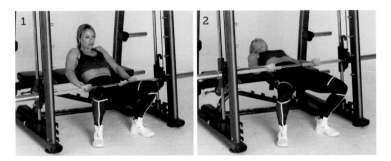

E 3 sets » 15 reps » 1 minute rest between sets

H 4 sets » 12 reps » 1 minute rest between sets

Deadlift with Olympic Bar
Heavy weight

Make sure the weight is the same each side – use clips if you need to. Place the bar in front of your feet. Stand up straight with your feet hip-width apart, toes pointing forwards. Keeping your back straight and bending only at the hips and knees, crouch down so your hands are able to reach the bar. Grasp the bar either side of your legs, placing one hand in an overhand grip and the other in an underhand grip (whichever is more comfortable is fine). Once you have a good grip, stand up straight, pushing down through your heels as you do so. As you come into a fully vertical standing position, squeeze your buttocks at the top of the movement. Keeping the bar against your legs, slowly allow it to pull you back down to the ground again, keeping your back straight and bending only at the hips and knees at all times. Allow the bar to hit the floor, take a breath and repeat the lift for the full amount of sets and reps.

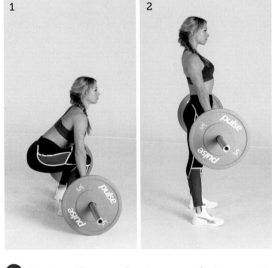

E 3 sets » 15 reps » 1 minute rest between sets

H 4 sets » 12 reps » 1 minute rest between sets

S 5 sets » 5 reps » 3 minutes rest between sets

Leg Curls on Machine
Heavy weight

Sit down on the machine, placing the backs of your ankles over the cushioned bar in front of you. You may need to adjust the chair so that your ankles sit comfortably on top of it. Slowly and gently push the cushioned bar down using your ankles and hamstrings. Then slowly and gently allow the bar to come back up to its starting position. Take a deep breath and repeat this movement for the full amount of sets and reps.

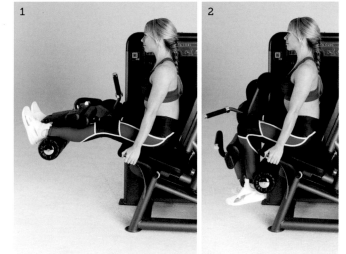

E 3 sets » 15 reps »
1 minute rest between sets

H 4 sets » 12 reps »
1 minute rest between sets

Leg Extension on Machine Heavy weight

Sit down on the machine, placing the fronts of your ankles under the cushioned bar in front of you. You may need to adjust the chair so that your ankles sit comfortably underneath it. Slowly and gently push the cushioned bar up using your ankles and quadriceps. Then slowly and gently allow the bar to come down to its starting position. Take a deep breath and repeat this movement for the full amount of sets and reps.

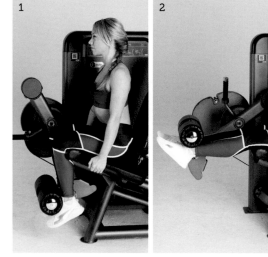

E 3 sets » 15 reps »
1 minute rest between sets

H 4 sets » 12 reps »
1 minute rest between sets

Tuesday + Friday Upper Body

Shoulder Press on Smith Machine
Heavy weight

Sit down and grab the handles with both hands. Push the handles up into the air and hold them there for a second before slowly bringing them back down. Repeat this movement for the full amount of sets and reps.

- **E** 3 sets » 15 reps » 1 minute rest between sets
- **H** 4 sets » 12 reps » 1 minute rest between sets
- **S** 5 sets » 5 reps » 3 minutes rest between sets

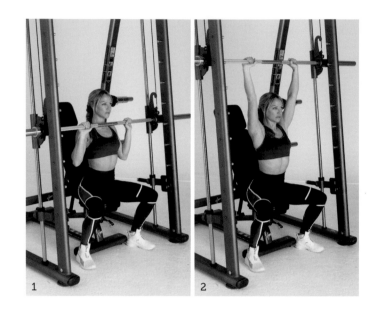

Lateral Raises on Cable Machine
Heavy weight

Attach the correct handle to the cable and make sure the weight you choose on the machine is appropriate (shoulders only need a light weight). With a slight bend in your elbow, and keeping your arm locked in this position, slowly raise the handle into the air until your arm is horizontal to your body. Allow the handle to pull your arm slowly back down into your starting position. Repeat the movement for the full amount of sets and reps on each arm.

- **E** 3 sets » 15 reps » 1 minute rest between sets
- **H** 4 sets » 12 reps » 1 minute rest between sets

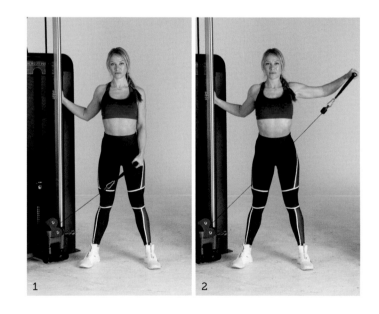

Front Raises on Cable Machine Heavy weight

Attach the correct handle to the cable and make sure the weight you choose on the machine is appropriate (shoulders usually need a very light weight). Grab the handle with an overhand grip. With a slight bend in your elbow, and keeping your arms locked in this position, slowly raise the handle up into the air out in front of you. Allow the handle to slowly pull your arms back down into your starting position. Repeat this movement for the full amount of sets and reps.

E 3 sets » 15 reps »
1 minute rest between sets

H 4 sets » 12 reps »
1 minute rest between sets

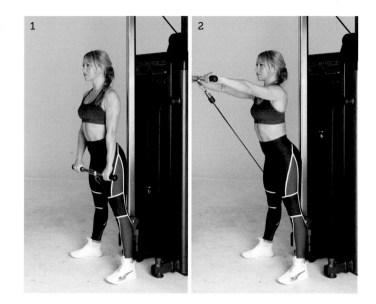

When it comes to the equipment you choose to use, switching it up between dumbbells, barbells, cables and static machinery is a really good idea. Doing this will continue to challenge and work your muscles in new and varied ways, as well as improve your overall strength, fitness, experience and enjoyment in the gym.

Tuesday + Friday Upper Body

Bent Over Rows with Olympic Bar *Heavy weight*

Stand up straight with your feet hip-width apart. Grab the bar with both hands and pull your shoulders back. Keeping an arch in your back and holding the bar against your lower body, slowly come down into a hamstring stretch until you have reached your full range of motion. Once there, pull the bar up into your ribcage, then slowly lower it back down again. Take a deep breath and repeat this movement for the full amount of sets and reps.

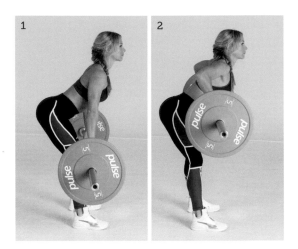

E 3 sets » 15 reps » 1 minute rest between sets

H 4 sets » 12 reps » 1 minute rest between sets

S 5 sets » 5 reps » 3 minutes rest between sets

Chest Press with Olympic Bar *Heavy weight*

(I would rather you use a bench press – a bench underneath a racked Olympic bar – for chest press exercises. However, if you have to use a Smith machine – illustrated here – that's fine.) Make sure the weight is the same each side of the bar – use clips if you need to. Lie back on the bench with your feet either side and flat on the floor. Reaching up, grip the bar with both hands – your hands should be directly above your shoulders. Push the bar up so it is free from the holding, then bring it down slowly so it lightly touches your chest. Push the bar back up into the air and hold it there for a second before bringing it back down. Repeat this movement for the full amount of sets and reps.

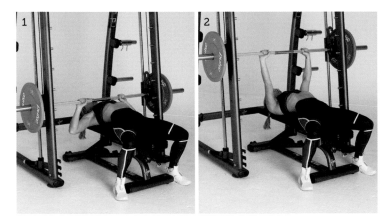

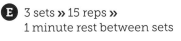

E 3 sets » 15 reps »
1 minute rest between sets

H 4 sets » 12 reps »
1 minute rest between sets

S 5 sets » 5 reps »
3 minutes rest between sets

SUPERSET

1 Bicep Curls
Heavy dumbbells

Stand up straight with your feet hip-width apart. Grip a dumbbell in each hand and allow them to hang either side of your hips. Keeping your arms in tight to your sides at all times, slowly lift the dumbbells from hip height into your shoulders, twisting the dumbbells into a horizontal position as you do so. Slowly lower the dumbbells back down to their starting position. Continue this movement for the full amount of sets and reps.

E 15 reps each arm   **H** 12 reps each arm

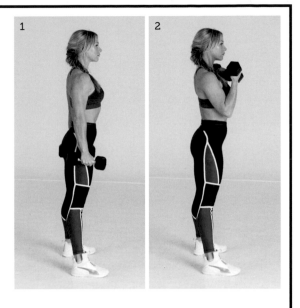

2 Tricep Extensions
Heavy dumbbell

Stand up straight with your feet close together. Grip the dumbbell with both hands and lift it into the air, holding it directly above your head. Bending only at the elbows, slowly allow the dumbbell to drop down behind you between your shoulder blades. Using your triceps, lift the dumbbell up back into the air above your head to your starting position. Repeat this movement for the full amount of sets and reps.

E 15 reps   **H** 12 reps

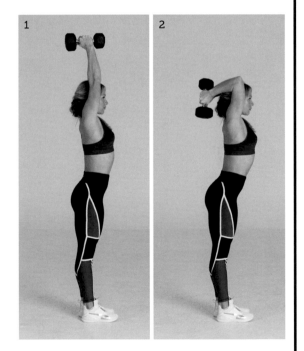

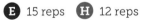

E 3 sets TOTAL 1 minute rest between sets   **H** 4 sets TOTAL 1 minute rest between sets

Wednesday + Saturday Back/Core

TRI SET

1 Wide Grip Pullups
Assisted

Make sure the padded seat is upright. Facing the machine, grip the bars that are furthest apart using an overhand grip and place your knees on top of the seat. Slowly allow your body to drop down underneath the bars. Once your arms are fully extended, slowly pull yourself back up into a wide-grip pull-up position. Hold this for a second before allowing yourself to come back down to your starting position. Take a deep breath and repeat this movement for the full amount of sets and reps.

E 15 reps   **H** 12 reps

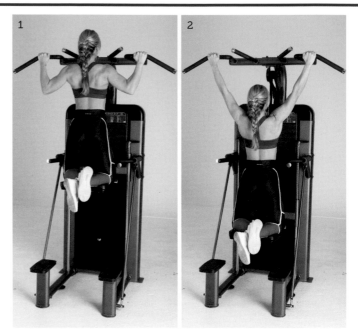

If your gym has an Assisted Machine, then that is perfect for this Tri Set. If not, simply tie a resistance band around a high bar and hook in your ankles or rest on your knees. You can then perform tricep dips on a bench or a bar.

2 Close Grip Pullups
Assisted

Make sure the padded seat is upright. Facing the machine, grip the bars that are closest together using an underhand grip. Place your knees on top of the seat, then slowly allow your body to drop down underneath the bars. Once your arms are fully extended, slowly pull yourself back up into a pull-up position. Hold this position for a second before allowing yourself to come back down again. Take a deep breath and repeat this movement for the full amount of sets and reps.

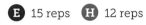 15 reps 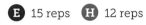 12 reps

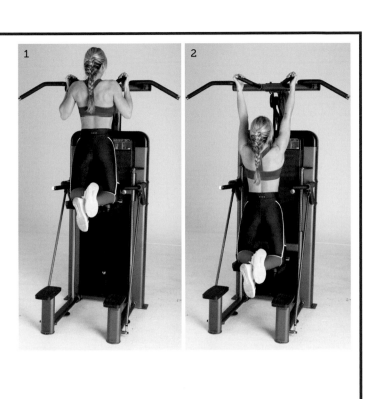

3 Tricep Dips Assisted

Make sure the padded seat is upright and the bars on either side of the machine are as close together as possible (they are often adjustable). Facing the machine, grip the bars and place your knees on top of the seat. Keeping your elbows in tight to your sides, slowly allow your body to drop down. When you have come down as far as possible, slowly push yourself back up, using your triceps. Take a deep breath and repeat this movement for the full amount of sets and reps.

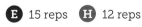 15 reps 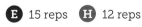 12 reps

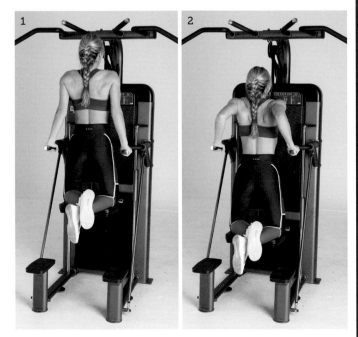

E 3 sets TOTAL 1 minute rest between sets H 4 sets TOTAL 1 minute rest between sets

Wednesday + Saturday Back/Core

★★ SUPERSET

1 Wide Grip Rows on Machine Heavy weight

You can do these on a static machine or using the cable machine (as illustrated), depending on what equipment your gym has. Either sit with your legs either side of the machine or stand with your feet together and knees bent. Holding the bar using an overhand grip, take a deep breath and slowly and gently pull the bar into your chest. Hold it against yourself for a second, then slowly and gently let it pull you back to the starting position. Take a deep breath and repeat this movement for the full amount of sets and reps.

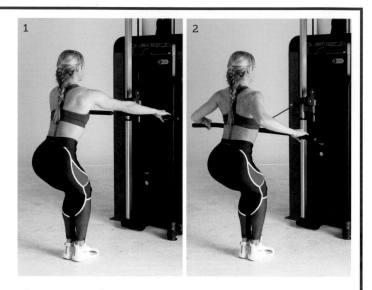

E 15 reps   **H** 12 reps

2 Close Grip Rows on Machine Heavy weight

You can do these on a static machine (as illustrated) or using the cable machine, depending on what equipment your gym has. Sit down with your legs either side of the machine and grip the handles in front of you with an inverted grip. Take a deep breath and, slowly and gently, pull the handles into your chest. Hold the handles against yourself for a second, then slowly and gently let them pull you back to the starting position. Take a deep breath and repeat this movement for the full amount of sets and reps.

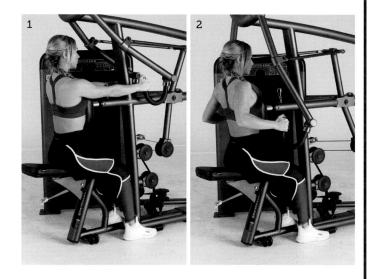

E 15 reps   **H** 12 reps

E 3 sets TOTAL 1 minute rest between sets   **H** 4 sets TOTAL 1 minute rest between sets

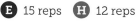

SUPERSET

1 Leg Raises on Machine
Unweighted

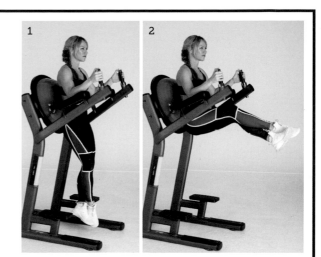

Stand on the machine. Keep your back straight against the back pad and grip both the handles. Let your legs dangle underneath you and cross your ankles. Slowly raise your legs up in front of you, then slowly allow them to come back down to your starting position. Repeat this movement fluidly to exhaust.

E 1 set to exhaust

H 1 set to exhaust

2 **The Plank** Unweighted

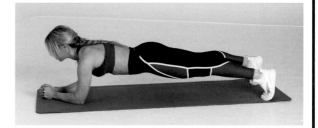

You may need a mat or cushion for your elbows during this exercise. Lie on your front with your feet hip-width apart. Rest on your elbows and keep your forearms flat against the mat. Make sure your elbows are underneath your shoulders. Pushing against your toes and forearms, raise your body up into an elevated plank. Do not allow your spine to curve, either concavely or convexly – you want a straight back. Hold this position to exhaust. If you are struggling, feel free to transfer your weight from one foot to another, essentially shuffling your feet while holding the plank position.

E 1 set to exhaust

H 1 set to exhaust

SUNDAY = FULL REST DAY

THE WEIGHT-TRAINING PLAN
Intermediate

Week 4 Aim to Increase
(aim to increase weights if/when possible)

Monday + Thursday = Lower Body

Tuesday + Friday = Upper Body

Wednesday + Saturday = Back/Core

Sunday = Rest day

You'll see this is a 6-day weight-lifting plan. However, you only need to train for 4 or 5 days a week, if you'd prefer.

As long as you make sure you train your body evenly – at least 1 day on your Lower Body, 1 day on your Upper Body and 1 day on your Back/Core – feel free to weight-train anywhere between 4 and 6 days a week, taking rest days as and when you need them.

Key to symbols

E Endurance

H Hypertrophy

S Strength. If Strength is your goal but the symbol is missing from an exercise, leave the exercise out.

Monday + Thursday Lower Body

Squats on Squat Rack with Olympic Bar Heavy weight

Make sure the weight is the same on either side – use clips if you need to. Find the centre of the horizontal bar and duck underneath it, so the bar is resting across your shoulders. Take hold of the bar either side of your shoulders and come up slightly on your tiptoes. Remove the bar from its holdings and take a few cautious steps backwards. Place your feet hip-width apart, or slightly further if that is a more comfortable position for you; make sure your toes are either pointing forwards or slightly outwards, whichever is more comfortable. Standing up straight and bending only at the hip and knees, come down into a low squat before pushing back up through your heels to a standing position, squeezing your glutes as you do so. Take a breath and repeat this movement for the full amount of sets and reps.

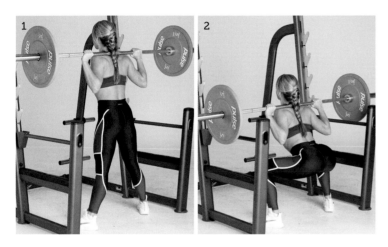

E 3 sets » 15 reps »
1 minute rest between sets

H 4 sets » 12 reps »
1 minute rest between sets

S INCREASE WEIGHT
3 sets » 3 reps »
3 minutes rest between sets

Deadlift with Olympic Bar
Heavy weight

Make sure the weight is the same each side – use clips if you need to. Place the bar in front of your feet. Stand up straight with your feet hip-width apart, toes pointing forwards. Keeping your back straight and bending only at the hips and knees, crouch down so your hands are able to reach the bar. Grasp the bar either side of your legs, placing one hand in an overhand grip and the other in an underhand grip (whichever is more comfortable is fine). Once you have a good grip, stand up straight, pushing down through your heels as you do so. As you come into a fully vertical standing position, squeeze your buttocks at the top of the movement. Keeping the bar against your legs, slowly allow it to pull you back down to the ground again, keeping your back straight and bending only at the hips and knees at all times. Allow the bar to hit the floor, take a breath and repeat the lift for the full amount of sets and reps.

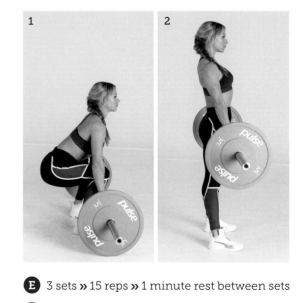

E 3 sets » 15 reps » 1 minute rest between sets

H 4 sets » 12 reps » 1 minute rest between sets

S INCREASE WEIGHT
3 sets » 3 reps » 3 minutes rest between sets

Monday + Thursday Lower Body

Leg Abductor on Machine Heavy weight

Sit up straight on the machine and make sure the weight is right for you. Place your knees inside the pads. Keeping your back fully straight, push the pads outwards with your knees. This movement may seem like a leg movement, but this really should be (and feel like) a sitting thrust. The movement should be coming from your hips, into your glutes. Repeat this movement for the full amount of sets and reps.

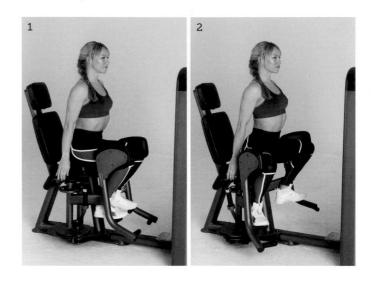

E 3 sets » 15 reps »
1 minute rest between sets

H 4 sets » 12 reps »
1 minute rest between sets

Hip **ab**ductors are your outside hip muscles, located around your upper glute area.

Hip **ad**ductors are inside hip muscles, located around your inner thighs (think of your legs coming or 'adding' together).

Leg Adductor on Machine Heavy weight

Sit up straight on the machine and make sure the weight is right for you. Place your knees outside the pads. Keeping your back fully straight, push the pads inwards with your knees. This movement may seem like a leg movement, but this really should be (and feel like) an inner thigh exercise. Repeat this movement for the full amount of sets and reps.

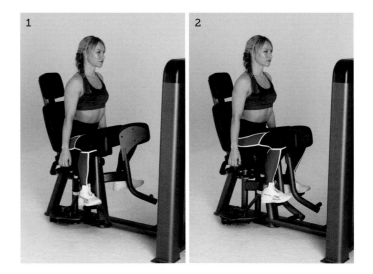

E 3 sets » 15 reps »
1 minute rest between sets

H 4 sets » 12 reps »
1 minute rest between sets

Donkey Kick Backs on Smith Machine OR Cable Machine
Heavy weight

Place a thick mat directly underneath the Smith bar. Make sure the weight is the same on each side of the bar. Kneel on the mat slightly in front of the bar and get down on all fours. Place the ball of your right foot under the bar and push up a little, then roll the bar back a little using the ball of your foot, and it will unhook itself. This needs a little skill and it may take a few sessions until you can do it seamlessly, but you will get there. Slowly and gently bring your knee down towards the mat and then push up until your leg is almost fully extended, always keeping a slight bend in the knee. Take a breath and repeat this movement for the full amount of sets and reps on each leg.

OR You can also do DKBs on the cable machine. Attach a Velcro ankle strap to the cable, stand upright and kick your leg back into the air while engaging your glute.

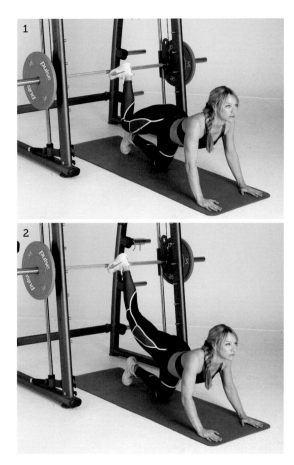

E 3 sets » 15 reps » 1 minute rest between sets

H 4 sets » 12 reps » 1 minute rest between sets

Hyperextensions on Machine
Heavy weight

(Please note that the illustration shows an unweighted hyperextension on the mat. If your gym has a hyperextension machine, though, this is preferable. Hold a weight plate against your chest as you do the hyperextensions on the machine.) Slowly bow your body back into a lower back crunch (another name for this exercise is a reverse sit up). Make sure you engage your glutes and core while doing this exercise. Hold this position for a few seconds then repeat the movement for the full amount of sets and reps.

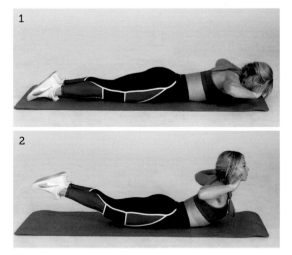

E 3 sets » 15 reps » 1 minute rest between sets

H 4 sets » 12 reps » 1 minute rest between sets

Tuesday + Friday Upper Body

TRI SET

1 Seated Military Press with Barbell Heavy barbell

Adjust the bench so it is upright. Grip the bar with your hands using an overhand grip, making sure they are shoulder-width apart. Resting the bar on top of your thighs, sit down on the bench, with your back fully upright against it and your feet on either side. Swing the bar up quickly so that it is at chest height. Push the bar up above your head until your arms are fully extended. Hold the bar above your head for a second, then slowly bring it back down to chest height. Take a deep breath and repeat this movement for the full amount of sets and reps.

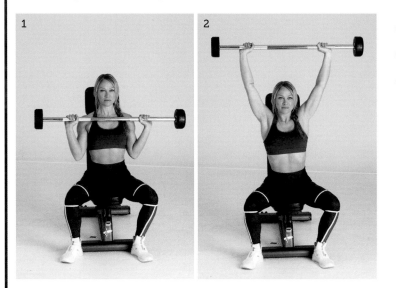

E 15 reps

H 12 reps

S INCREASE WEIGHT
3 sets » 3 reps »
3 minutes rest between sets

Super Sets and Tri Sets will have you struggling after the first exercise. If you have to lower the weight a little in order to complete the full sets and reps, that's absolutely fine; just make sure you are still challenging yourself throughout!

2 Lateral Raises
Heavy dumbbells

Make sure the weight is the same in each hand. Stand up straight with your knees slightly bent and your feet together. Grip the dumbbells in front of your crotch, lightly touching each other. Lean ever-so-slightly forward with your upper body, keeping a slight arch in your lower back. Keeping a slight bend in your elbows and bowing them outwards slightly, slowly and gradually raise the dumbbells out either side of you, until your arms are horizontal, like an eagle in flight. Hold this position for a fraction of a second, then slowly bring your arms back down to your starting position. Take a breath and repeat this movement for the full amount of sets and reps.

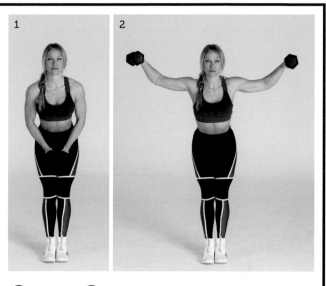

E 15 reps **H** 12 reps

3 Front Raises
Heavy dumbbells

Make sure the weight is the same in each hand. Stand up straight with your feet hip-width apart and your toes pointing forwards. Grip the dumbbells horizontally, using an overhand grip, and allow them to hang together in front of your crotch. Keeping your back straight at all times, take a deep breath and slowly raise one of the dumbbells. Keep a slight bend in your elbow as you do so. Hold the dumbbell in its raised position for a fraction of a second, then slowly bring it back down. Repeat with the other arm. Continue this movement alternately for the full amount of sets and reps.

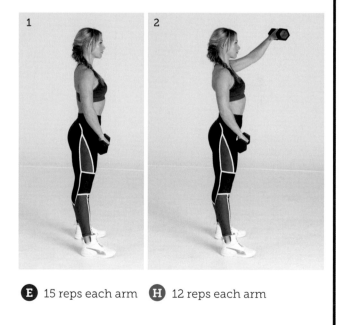

E 15 reps each arm **H** 12 reps each arm

E 3 sets TOTAL 1 minute rest between sets **H** 4 sets TOTAL 1 minute rest between sets

Tuesday + Friday Upper Body

Bent Over Rows with Olympic Bar Heavy weight

Stand up straight with your feet hip-width apart. Grab the bar with both hands and pull your shoulders back. Keeping an arch in your back and holding the bar against your lower body, slowly come down into a hamstring stretch until you have reached your full range of motion. Once there, pull the bar up into your ribcage, then slowly lower it back down again. Take a deep breath and repeat this movement for the full amount of sets and reps.

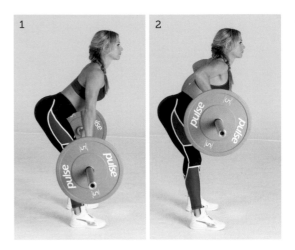

E 3 sets » 15 reps » 1 minute rest between sets

H 4 sets » 12 reps » 1 minute rest between sets

S 3 sets » 3 reps » 3 minutes rest between sets

Chest Press with Olympic Bar Heavy weight

(I would rather you use a bench press – a bench underneath a racked Olympic bar – for chest press exercises. However, if you have to use a Smith machine – illustrated here – that's fine.) Make sure the weight is the same each side of the bar – use clips if you need to. Lie back on the bench with your feet either side and flat on the floor. Reaching up, grip the bar with both your hands – your hands should be directly above your shoulders. Push the bar up so it is free from the holding, then bring it down slowly so it lightly touches your chest. Push the bar back up into the air and hold it there for a second before bringing it back down. Repeat this movement for the full amount of sets and reps.

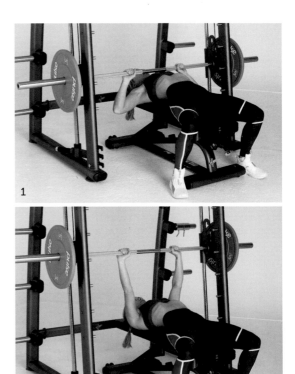

E 3 sets » 15 reps » 1 minute rest between sets

H 4 sets » 12 reps » 1 minute rest between sets

S **INCREASE WEIGHT**
3 sets » 3 reps » 3 minutes rest between sets

SUPERSET

1 Bicep Curls
Heavy dumbbells

Stand up straight with your feet hip-width apart. Grip a dumbbell in each hand and allow them to hang either side of your hips. Keeping your arms in tight to your sides at all times, slowly lift the dumbbells from hip height into your shoulders, twisting the dumbbells into a horizontal position as you do so. Slowly lower the dumbbells back down to their starting position. Repeat on the opposite arm. Continue this movement for the full amount of sets and reps.

E 15 reps each arm   **H** 12 reps each arm

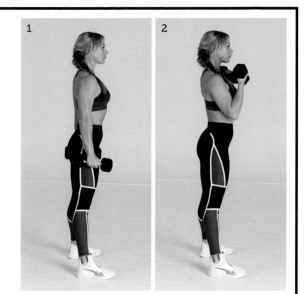

2 Tricep Extensions
Heavy dumbbell

Stand up straight with your feet close together. Grip the dumbbell with both hands and lift it into the air, holding it directly above your head. Bending only at the elbows, slowly allow the dumbbell to drop down behind you between your shoulder blades. Using your triceps, lift the dumbbell up back into the air above your head to your starting position. Repeat this movement for the full amount of sets and reps.

E 15 reps   **H** 12 reps

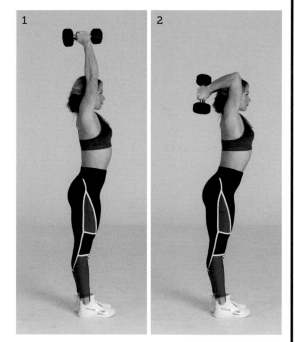

E 3 sets TOTAL 1 minute rest between sets   **H** 4 sets TOTAL 1 minute rest between sets

Wednesday + Saturday Back/Core

★★ **SUPERSET**

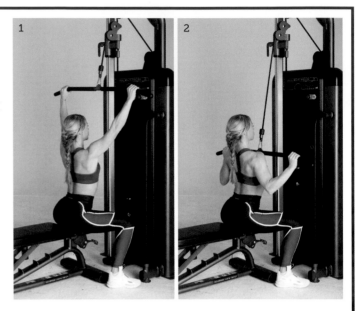

1 Wide Grip Pulldowns on Machine Heavy weight

You can do this on a specific cable machine with a bench attached, or you can improvise as I have done in the illustration, by pulling a bench up close to any cable machine. Attach the long bar to the cable machine and make sure it's at its highest setting. Sit down on the bench, fully upright, and grab the bar on either side of the cable with an overhand grip. Pull the bar down in front of your chest and slowly let it pull your arms back up again. Repeat this movement for the full amount of sets and reps.

E 15 reps   **H** 12 reps

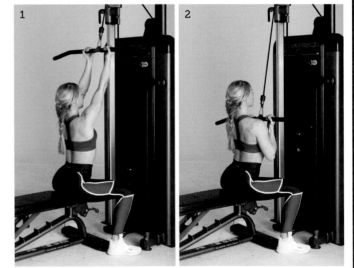

2 Close Grip Pulldowns on Machine Heavy weight

You can do this on a specific cable machine with a bench attached, or you can improvise, as I have done in the illustration, by pulling a bench up close to any cable machine. Attach any bar to the cable machine and make sure it's at its highest setting. Sit down on the bench, fully upright, and grab the bar on either side of the cable with an underhand grip. Pull the bar down in front of your chest and slowly let it pull your arms back up again. Repeat this movement for the full amount of sets and reps.

E 15 reps   **H** 12 reps

E 3 sets TOTAL 1 minute rest between sets   **H** 4 sets TOTAL 1 minute rest between sets

SUPERSET

1 Wide Grip Rows on Machine Heavy weight

You can do these on a static machine or using the cable machine (as illustrated), depending on what equipment your gym has. Either sit with your legs either side of the machine or stand with your feet together and knees bent. Holding the bar using an overhand grip, take a deep breath and slowly and gently pull the bar into your chest. Hold it against yourself for a second, then slowly and gently let it pull you back to the starting position. Take a deep breath and repeat this movement for the full amount of sets and reps.

E 15 reps **H** 12 reps

2 Close Grip Rows on Machine Heavy weight

You can do these on a static machine (as illustrated) or using the cable machine, depending on what equipment your gym has. Sit down with your legs either side of the machine and grip the handles in front of you with an inverted grip. Take a deep breath and, slowly and gently, pull the handles into your chest. Hold the handles against yourself for a second, then slowly and gently let them pull you back to the starting position. Take a deep breath and repeat this movement for the full amount of sets and reps.

E 15 reps **H** 12 reps

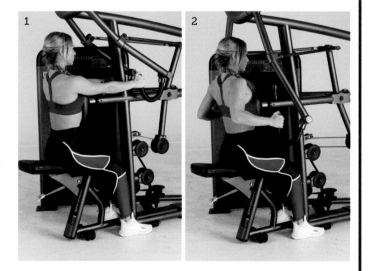

E 3 sets TOTAL 1 minute rest between sets   **H** 4 sets TOTAL 1 minute rest between sets

Wednesday + Saturday Back/Core

 SUPERSET

1 Leg Raises on Machine
Unweighted

Stand on the machine. Keep your back straight against the back pad and grip both the handles. Let your legs dangle underneath you and cross your ankles. Slowly raise your legs up in front of you, then slowly allow them to come back down to your starting position. Repeat this movement fluidly to exhaust.

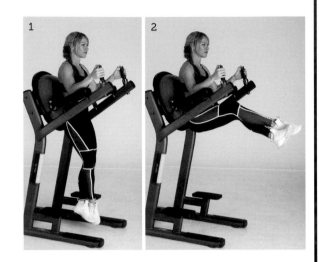

E 1 set to exhaust

H 1 set to exhaust

2 The Plank Unweighted

You may need a mat or cushion for your elbows during this exercise. Lie on your front with your feet hip-width apart. Rest on your elbows and keep your forearms flat against the mat. Make sure your elbows are underneath your shoulders. Pushing against your toes and forearms, raise your body up into an elevated plank. Do not allow your spine to curve, either concavely or convexly – you want a straight back. Hold this position to exhaust. If you are struggling, feel free to transfer your weight from one foot to another, essentially shuffling your feet while holding the plank position.

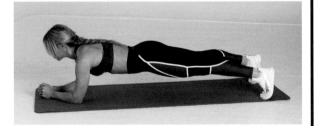

E 1 set to exhaust

H 1 set to exhaust

SUNDAY = FULL REST DAY

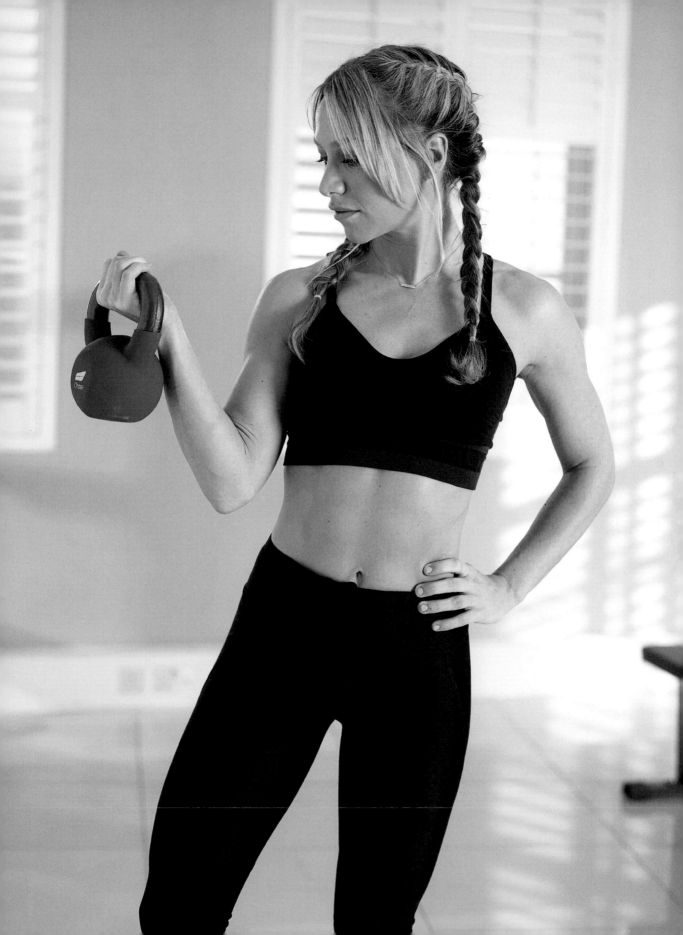

ADVANCED

This section is for those of you who know how to lift and have been lifting for a while. However, please be aware that it isn't going to turn you into someone who can flip a tyre as you catch a dumbbell and bicep curl a donkey for 100 sets of 100 reps.

There is a weird idea in the weight-lifting world that the more advanced you are, the more complicated your programme becomes... As far as I'm concerned, as both a Personal Trainer and a long-term lifter, this is absolute nonsense. The four staple exercises of any good lifting plan should always be:

» Squats
» Deadlifts
» Rows
» Presses

These big, compound, push/pull movements are going to hit your body in multiple ways that other, more isolated exercises will not. But there is a time and a place for more isolated work, and you will see that in this section, too.

What is different about the Advanced Plan is that I now encourage you to really *push* your lifting...

Whether this be in terms of your:

» Work rate – are you really working hard and pushing yourself in every session?
» Volume – should you be progressively adding sets and / or reps?
» Intensity – should you try to increase the weight you are lifting?

Are you really giving your training the 110% that only an advanced lifter can give?

While I do want you to really push yourself, never forget that form is ALWAYS primary, weight is ALWAYS secondary. **There is no point in lifting heavy if you can't lift *properly*.**

Choosing Your Weight-Training Goal

» **Endurance Training** (*the muscle's ability to generate force repeatedly*) is perfect for those wanting to increase their 'functional' training abilities, such as triathletes, distance runners and rowers. If you are a cardio bunny looking to implement some weight lifting to assist your sport, then endurance is perfect for you.

» **Hypertrophy Training** (*the growth of a muscle*) is perfect for those wanting to increase visible muscle mass, and is my favourite form of weight lifting. If you are looking for aesthetic muscular results, hypertrophy is for you.

» **Strength Training** (*the muscle's ability to generate force against resistance*) or powerlifting is perfect for those wanting to increase their physical strength and really enjoy their weight lifting. It traditionally only calls for 3 exercises – squat, deadlift and bench press, as these are the competition lifts. However, in recent years 2 common exercises have been included in the training – military press and barbell row.

No matter what your goal (endurance, hypertrophy or strength), form should *always* be primary, weight secondary.

I have written the exercise plans to cover all the bases so there are 2 days for each different area of the body (upper, lower and back / core). As a result, each plan has 6 days a week of training BUT you do not need to train for the full 6 days. As long as you train your body evenly (don't just focus on legs, for example), feel free to weight-train anywhere between 4 and 6 times a week, taking rest days as and when you need them. This advice is especially important with strength training – recovery is key for this goal, so training 4 days a week is enough.

Try not to train the same body part 2 days in a row, as you want to make sure each muscle group has at least 24 hours to recover after training.

When I instruct a *Heavy Weight*, I mean a weight that challenges you to really push HARD by your last few reps.

You can continue to use this plan for up to 24 weeks (6 months) in total. Progress in terms of increasing weight and / or sets and reps whenever and wherever possible and your results will improve and increase week on week.

After that 24-week (6-month) mark, I recommend that you think about switching up your plan, whether that is in terms of the specific exercises you are doing, your training zone (endurance/hypertrophy/strength), volume (sets and reps), intensity (weight), or simply diversifying what you're doing for a period of time.

I try to implement a new lifting plan twice a year and I credit this tactic with not only continuing to grow my muscle, but also increasing my experience and helping me learn what exercises do and don't work best for me.

If you consider yourself an advanced lifter, I want you to really push yourself hard when you train. If you know you can increase your volume or intensity, front up and do it! If you hit a wall with your training, switch up your training zone for a week and try to break through the plateau.

Advanced

> **Week 1** Overload Focused
> *(increased weight / volume / intensity)*
>
> Monday + Thursday = Lower Body
>
> Tuesday + Friday = Upper Body
>
> Wednesday + Saturday = Back/Core
>
> Sunday = Rest day

You'll see this is a 6-day weight-lifting plan. However, you only need to train for 4 or 5 days a week, if you'd prefer.

As long as you make sure you train your body evenly – at least 1 day on your Lower Body, 1 day on your Upper Body and 1 day on your Back/Core – feel free to weight-train anywhere between 4 and 6 days a week, taking rest days as and when you need them.

Key to symbols

E Endurance

H Hypertrophy

S Strength. If Strength is your goal but the symbol is missing from an exercise, leave the exercise out.

Monday + Thursday Lower Body

Wide Stance Squats on Squat Rack Heavy weight

Make sure the weight is the same on either side of the bar – use clips if you need to. Find the centre of the horizontal bar and duck underneath it, so the bar is resting across your shoulders. Take hold of the bar either side of your shoulders and, coming up slightly on your tiptoes, remove the bar from its holdings and take a few cautious steps backwards. Place your feet slightly further than hip-width apart and make sure your toes are either pointing forwards or slightly outwards, whichever is more comfortable. When you have your position right and you are ready standing up straight, come down into a low squat, bending only at the hips and knees, before pushing back up through your heels to a standing position, squeezing your glutes as you do so. Take a breath and repeat this movement for the full amount of sets and reps.

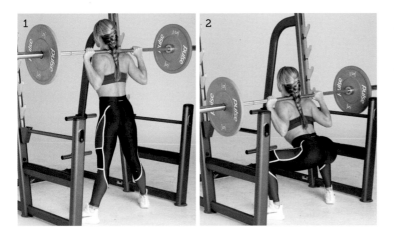

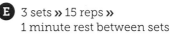

E 3 sets **»** 15 reps **»** 1 minute rest between sets

H 4 sets **»** 12 reps **»** 1 minute rest between sets

S 5 sets **»** 5 reps **»** 3 minutes rest between sets

Bulgarian Split Squats on Smith Machine Heavy weight

Place the bench about 0.5m behind you. Find the centre of the horizontal bar and duck underneath it, so the bar is resting across your shoulders. Place one foot up on the bench behind you, resting top down. Make sure the toes of your standing foot are pointing forwards. Take hold of the bar either side of your shoulders and unhook the bar from the machine – keep it unhooked using your grip. Standing up straight and bending only at the hip and knee, come down into a low squat before pushing back up through your heel to a standing position. Take a breath and repeat on the other leg. Repeat for the full amount of sets and reps.

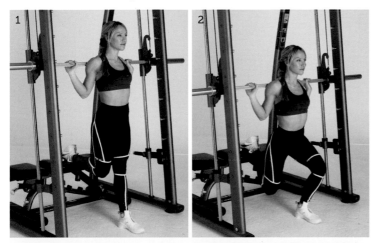

E 3 sets **»** 15 reps **»** 1 minute rest between sets

H 4 sets **»** 12 reps **»** 1 minute rest between sets

Monday + Thursday Lower Body

Hip Thrusts on Smith Machine Heavy weight

(Please note: the illustration shows the machine unweighted – this exercise should be weighted.) Place a bench about 0.5m behind you, so you are sandwiched between the Smith and the bench. Lower the bar so it is about 30cm off the ground. Sit down on the floor between the bar and the bench, facing the bar and resting your upper back and shoulder blades on the edge of the bench. Place a bar pad (a black, cushioned tube) around the centre of the horizontal bar. Place your feet hip-width apart and keep your toes pointing forwards or slightly outwards. Place your hips underneath the bar and your hands either side of your hips. Unhook the bar from the machine – keep it unhooked using your grip – and thrust up into the air, through your glutes, squeezing them tight at the top of the movement. Hold this position for a few seconds before coming back down until your buttocks are just above the ground. Take a breath and repeat the movement for the full amount of sets and reps.

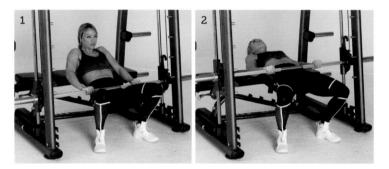

E 3 sets » 15 reps »
1 minute rest between sets

H 4 sets » 12 reps »
1 minute rest between sets

Deadlift with Olympic Bar
Heavy weight

Make sure the weight is the same each side – use clips if you need to. Place the bar in front of your feet. Stand up straight with your feet hip-width apart, toes pointing forwards. Keeping your back straight and bending only at the hips and knees, crouch down so your hands are able to reach the bar. Grasp the bar either side of your legs, placing one hand in an overhand grip and the other in an underhand grip (whichever is more comfortable is fine). Once you have a good grip, stand up straight, pushing down through your heels as you do so. As you come into a fully vertical standing position, squeeze your buttocks at the top of the movement. Keeping the bar against your legs, slowly allow it to pull you back down to the ground again, keeping your back straight and bending only at the hips and knees at all times. Allow the bar to hit the floor, take a breath and repeat the lift for the full amount of sets and reps.

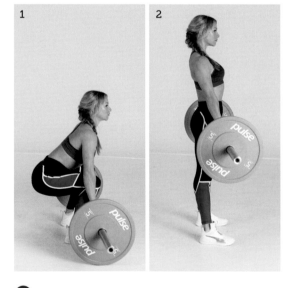

E 3 sets » 15 reps » 1 minute rest between sets

H 4 sets » 12 reps » 1 minute rest between sets

S 5 sets » 5 reps » 3 minutes rest between sets

Romanian Deadlift with Olympic Bar Heavy weight

Make sure the weight is the same each side – use clips if you need to. Place the bar in front of your feet. Stand up straight with your feet hip-width apart and your toes pointing forwards. Keeping your back straight and bending only at the hips and knees, crouch down so your hands are now able to grasp the bar. Grasp it either side of your legs, placing one hand in an overhand grip, the other in an underhand grip (whichever hand is more comfortable is fine). Once you have a good grip on the bar, stand up straight, pushing down through your heels as you do so. As you come into a full standing position, squeeze your buttocks at the top of the movement. Pull your shoulders back and keep them back during this exercise. Engage your core and make sure to keep your entire core and back position solid throughout. Keeping the bar against your legs, slowly allow it to pull you down from the hips as far as your hamstrings will allow – sticking your bottom out as you go. Take a breath and return to your starting position. Repeat the lift for the full amount of sets and reps.

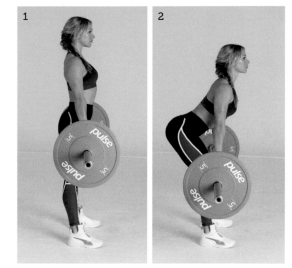

E 3 sets » 15 reps » 1 minute rest between sets

H 4 sets » 12 reps » 1 minute rest between sets

Leg Press on Machine
Heavy weight

Sit down and place your feet hip-width apart on the plate in front of you (or slightly further apart if that is more comfortable). Point your toes upwards, or slightly outwards. Pushing through the flats of your feet, slowly and gently push against the plate. Depending on the machine, the force will either push the plate away from your seat, or your seat away from the plate. When you have fully extended (without locking your knees out – you should always keep a slight bend in them when performing a lower body lift), slowly come back into your starting position. Take a breath and repeat this movement for the full amount of sets and reps. Finish with light calf presses to exhaust.

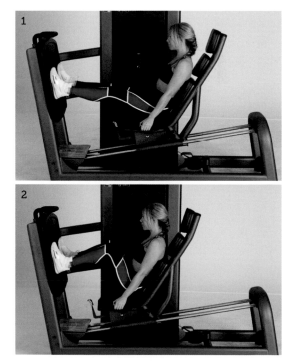

E 3 sets » 15 reps » 1 minute rest between sets

H 4 sets » 12 reps » 1 minute rest between sets

Tuesday + Friday Upper Body

TRI SET

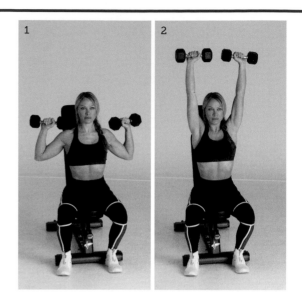

1 Seated Dumbbell Press
Heavy dumbbells

Adjust the bench so it's upright then sit up straight on the bench with your back against it. Hold a dumbbell in each hand and rest them on top of your thighs if need be. Bring them up to shoulder height and hold them horizontally. Push both dumbbells up into the air and gently touch them together at the top of the movement. Slowly bring them back down to shoulder height and repeat the movement for the full sets and reps.

E 15 reps   **H** 12 reps

S 5 sets » 5 reps » 3 minutes rest between sets

2 Lateral Raises
Heavy dumbbells

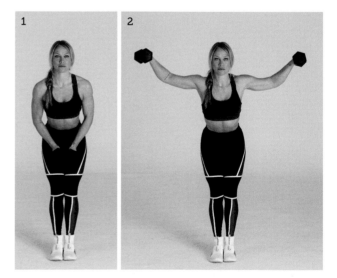

Make sure the weight is the same in each hand. Stand up straight with your knees slightly bent and your feet together. Grip the dumbbells in front of your crotch, lightly touching each other. Lean ever-so-slightly forward with your upper body, keeping a slight arch in your lower back. Keeping a slight bend in your elbows and bowing them outwards slightly, slowly and gradually raise the dumbbells out either side of you, until your arms are horizontal, like an eagle in flight. Hold this position for a fraction of a second, then slowly bring your arms back down to your starting position. Take a breath and repeat this movement for the full amount of sets and reps.

E 15 reps   **H** 12 reps

3 Front Raises Heavy dumbbells

Make sure the weight is the same in each hand. Stand up straight with your feet hip-width apart and your toes pointing forwards. Grip the dumbbells horizontally, using an overhand grip, and allow them to hang together in front of your crotch. Keeping your back straight at all times, take a deep breath and slowly raise one of the dumbbells. Keep a slight bend in your elbow as you do so. Hold the dumbbell in its raised position for a fraction of a second, then slowly bring it back down. Repeat with the other arm. Continue this movement alternately for the full amount of sets and reps.

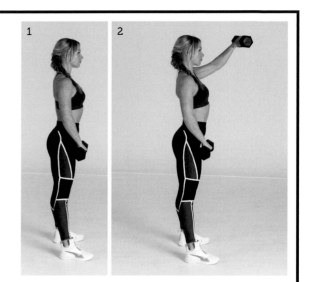

E 15 reps   **H** 12 reps

E 3 sets TOTAL 1 minute rest between sets   **H** 4 sets TOTAL 1 minute rest between sets

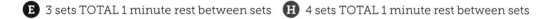

Tri Sets are hard but they are a great time saver and I find them really enjoyable. This kind of volume is a great way to fully exhaust the muscle. And if you are looking for a depletion workout, Super Sets, Tri Sets and Giant Sets are ideal.

Tuesday + Friday Upper Body

Bent Over Rows with Olympic Bar Heavy weight

Stand up straight with your feet hip-width apart. Grab the bar with both hands and pull your shoulders back. Keeping an arch in your back and holding the bar against your lower body, slowly come down into a hamstring stretch until you have reached your full range of motion. Once there, pull the bar up into your ribcage, then slowly lower it back down again. Take a deep breath and repeat this movement for the full amount of sets and reps.

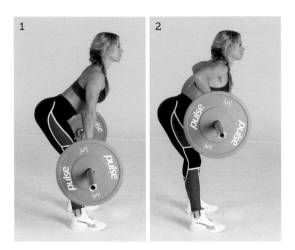

E 3 sets » 15 reps » 1 minute rest between sets

H 4 sets » 12 reps » 1 minute rest between sets

S 5 sets » 5 reps » 3 minutes rest between sets

Chest Press with Olympic Bar Heavy weight

(I would rather you use a bench press – a bench underneath a racked Olympic bar – for chest press exercies. However, if you have to use a Smith machine – illustrated here – that's fine.) Make sure the weight is the same each side – use clips if you need to. Lie back on the bench with your feet either side and flat on the floor. Reaching up, grip the bar with both hands – your hands should be directly above your shoulders. Push the bar up so it is free from the holding, then bring it down slowly so it lightly touches your chest. Push the bar back up into the air and hold it there for a second before bringing it back down. Repeat this movement for the full amount of sets and reps.

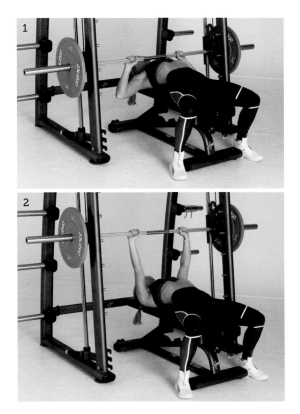

E 3 sets » 15 reps » 1 minute rest between sets

H 4 sets » 12 reps » 1 minute rest between sets

S 5 sets » 5 reps » 3 minutes rest between sets

Chest Fly on Bench
Heavy dumbbells

Make sure the weight is the same in each hand. Sit on the bench with your feet flat on the floor on either side and grip the dumbbells in your hands, resting them on top of your thighs. Lie down on the bench. Extend your arms out either side of your body at chest height. Then, as if you are hugging a beach ball, and keeping a slight bend in your elbows, bring the dumbbells together above your body. Slowly bring the dumbbells back down to the starting position. Take a breath and repeat this movement for the full amount of sets and reps.

E 3 sets » 15 reps » 1 minute rest between sets

H 4 sets » 12 reps » 1 minute rest between sets

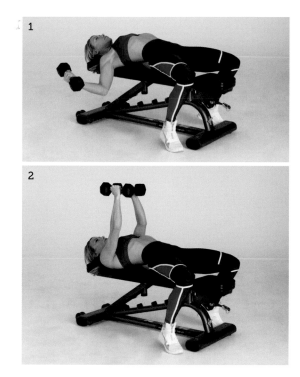

If you are strength training, taking time to recover between sets is pivotal. However, if you are in an endurance or hypertrophy training zone, take a minute to recover but, as soon as you feel able to go again, do. Don't waste time in the gym; you are there to work hard.

Wednesday + Saturday Back/Core

Hyperextensions on Machine
Heavy weight

(Please note that the illustration shows an unweighted hyperextension on the mat. If your gym has a hyperextension machine, though, this is preferable. Hold a weight plate against your chest as you do the hyperextensions on the machine.) Slowly bow your body back into a lower back crunch (another name for this exercise is a reverse sit up). Make sure you engage your glutes and core while doing this exercise. Hold this position for a few seconds then repeat this movement for the full amount of sets and reps.

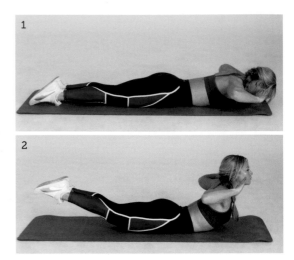

(E) 3 sets » 15 reps » 1 minute rest between sets

(H) 4 sets » 12 reps » 1 minute rest between sets

Dumbbell Pullovers on Bench
Heavy dumbbell

Sit on the bench, legs either side of it, and grip the dumbbell (vertically) between your legs. Lie down and, as you do so, raise the dumbbell up in the air, directly above your face. Now adjust your grip by opening your hands, allowing the weight of the dumbbell to rest against the flats of your palms, gripping around its base with your fingers. Allow the dumbbell to slowly and gently come behind you, so that it is behind your head and behind the bench. Slowly and gently bring it back up into the air, above your face, into your starting position. Take a deep breath and repeat this movement for the full amount of sets and reps.

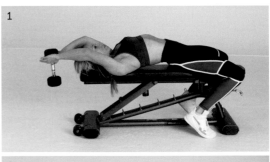

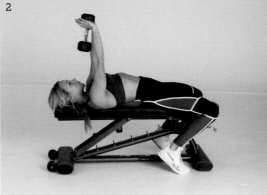

(E) 3 sets » 15 reps » 1 minute rest between sets

(H) 4 sets » 12 reps » 1 minute rest between sets

★★ SUPERSET

1 Wide Grip Rows on Machine Heavy weight

You can do these on a static machine or using the cable machine (as illustrated), depending on what equipment your gym has. Either sit with your legs either side of the machine or stand with your feet together and knees bent. Holding the bar using an overhand grip, take a deep breath and slowly and gently pull the bar into your chest. Hold it against yourself for a second, then slowly and gently let it pull you back to the starting position. Take a deep breath and repeat this movement for the full amount of sets and reps.

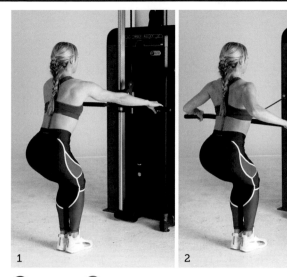

E 15 reps **H** 12 reps

2 Close Grip Rows on Machine Heavy weight

You can do these on a static machine (as illustrated) or using the cable machine, depending on what equipment your gym has. Sit down with your legs either side of the machine and grip the handles in front of you with an inverted grip. Take a deep breath and, slowly and gently, pull the handles into your chest. Hold the handles against yourself for a second, then slowly and gently let them pull you back to the starting position. Take a deep breath and repeat this movement for the full amount of sets and reps.

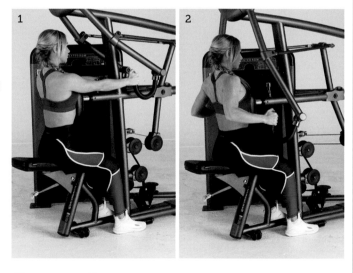

E 15 reps **H** 12 reps

E 3 sets TOTAL 1 minute rest between sets **H** 4 sets TOTAL 1 minute rest between sets

WEEK
1

Wednesday + Saturday Back/Core

Wide Grip Pullups on Machine Assisted

Make sure the padded seat is upright. Facing the machine, grip the bars that are furthest apart using an overhand grip and place your knees on top of the seat. Slowly allow your body to drop down underneath the bars. Once your arms are fully extended, slowly pull yourself back up into a wide-grip pull-up position. Hold this for a second before allowing yourself to come back down to your starting position. Take a deep breath and repeat this movement for the full amount of sets and reps.

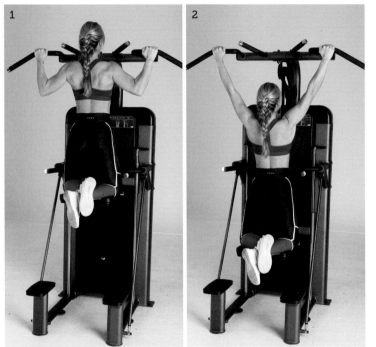

E 3 sets » 15 reps »
1 minute rest between sets

H 4 sets » 12 reps »
1 minute rest between sets

OR Unassisted

Grip the bars that are furthest apart using an overhand grip. Slowly allow your body to drop down underneath the bars and then swiftly pull yourself back up. Take a deep breath and repeat this movement for the full amount of sets and reps.

E 3 sets to exhaust » 1 minute rest between sets

H 4 sets to exhaust » 1 minute rest between sets

Close Grip Pullups on Machine Assisted

Make sure the padded seat is upright. Facing the machine, grip the bars above you that are closest together using an underhand grip. Place your knees on top of the seat, then slowly allow your body to drop down underneath the bars. Once your arms are fully extended, slowly pull yourself back up into a pull-up position. Hold this position for a second before allowing yourself to come back down again. Take a deep breath and repeat this movement for the full amount of sets and reps.

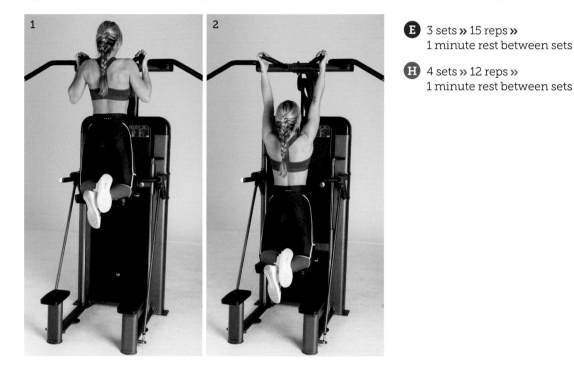

E 3 sets » 15 reps »
1 minute rest between sets

H 4 sets » 12 reps »
1 minute rest between sets

OR Unassisted

Grip the bars above you that are closest together using an underhand grip. Allow your body to drop down underneath the bars then swiftly pull yourself back up again. Take a deep breath and repeat this movement for the full amount of sets and reps.

E 3 sets to exhaust » 1 minute rest between sets

H 4 sets to exhaust » 1 minute rest between sets

SUNDAY = FULL REST DAY

Week 2 Overload Focused
(increased weight / volume / intensity)

Monday + Thursday = Lower Body

Tuesday + Friday = Upper Body

Wednesday + Saturday = Back/Core

Sunday = Rest day

You'll see this is a 6-day weight-lifting plan. However, you only need to train for 4 or 5 days a week, if you'd prefer.

As long as you make sure you train your body evenly – at least 1 day on your Lower Body, 1 day on your Upper Body and 1 day on your Back/Core – feel free to weight-train anywhere between 4 and 6 days a week, taking rest days as and when you need them.

Key to symbols

E Endurance

H Hypertrophy

S Strength. If Strength is your goal but the symbol is missing from an exercise, leave the exercise out.

Monday + Thursday Lower Body

Squats on Squat Rack with Olympic Bar Heavy weight

Make sure the weight is the same each side – use clips if you need to. Find the centre of the horizontal bar and duck underneath it, so the bar is resting across your shoulders. Take hold of the bar either side of your shoulders and come up slightly on your tiptoes. Remove the bar from its holdings and take a few cautious steps backwards. Place your feet hip-width apart, or slightly further if that is a more comfortable squat position for you, and make sure your toes are either pointing forwards or slightly outwards, whichever is more comfortable. Standing up straight and bending only at the hip and knees, come down into a low squat before pushing back up through your heels to a standing position, squeezing your glutes as you do so. Take a breath and repeat this movement for the full amount of sets and reps.

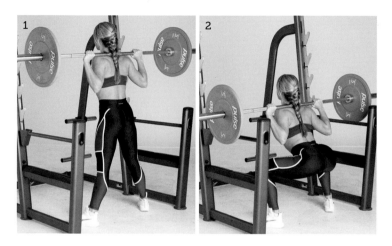

E 3 sets » 15 reps » 1 minute rest between sets

H 4 sets » 12 reps » 1 minute rest between sets

S 5 sets » 5 reps » 3 minutes rest between sets

Deadlift with Olympic Bar
Heavy weight

Make sure the weight is the same each side – use clips if you need to. Place the bar in front of your feet. Stand up straight with your feet hip-width apart, toes pointing forwards. Keeping your back straight and bending only at the hips and knees, crouch down so your hands are able to reach the bar. Grasp the bar either side of your legs, placing one hand in an overhand grip and the other in an underhand grip (whichever is more comfortable). Once you have a good grip, stand up straight, pushing down through your heels as you do so. As you come into a fully vertical standing position, squeeze your buttocks at the top of the movement. Keeping the bar against your legs, slowly allow it to pull you back down to the ground again, keeping your back straight and bending only at the hips and knees at all times. Allow the bar to hit the floor, take a breath and repeat the lift for the full amount of sets and reps.

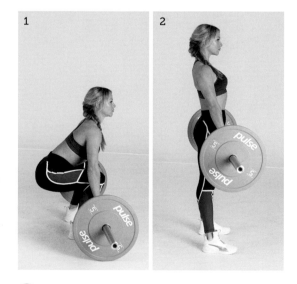

E 3 sets » 15 reps » 1 minute rest between sets

H 4 sets » 12 reps » 1 minute rest between sets

S 5 sets » 5 reps » 3 minutes rest between sets

Monday + Thursday Lower Body

Overhead Squats on Squat Rack with Olympic Bar
Heavy weight

(Please note: the illustration shows the bar unweighted – this exercise should be weighted.) Remove the bar from its holdings by gripping it in your hands and holding it tight against your chest. Take a few cautious steps backwards. Place your feet hip-width apart, or slightly further if that is a more comfortable squat position for you, and make sure your toes are either pointing forwards or slightly outwards, whichever is more comfortable. Push the bar up into the air above your head as you stand up straight. Come down into a low squat bending only at the hip and knees, before pushing back up through your heels to a standing position, squeezing your glutes as you do so. Take a breath and repeat this movement for the full amount of sets and reps.

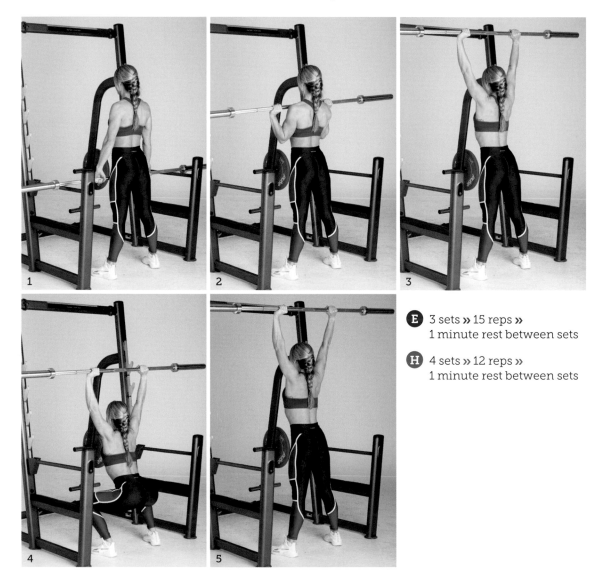

E 3 sets » 15 reps »
1 minute rest between sets

H 4 sets » 12 reps »
1 minute rest between sets

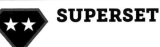 **SUPERSET**

1 Leg Curl on Machine
Heavy weight

Sit down on the machine, placing the backs of your ankles over the cushioned bar in front of you. You may need to adjust the chair so that your ankles sit comfortably on top of it. Slowly and gently push the cushioned bar down using your ankles and hamstrings. Then slowly and gently allow the bar to come back up to its starting position. Take a deep breath and repeat this movement for the full amount of sets and reps.

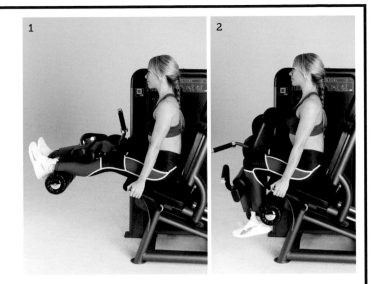

E 15 reps   **H** 12 reps

2 Leg Extension on Machine Heavy weight

Sit down on the machine, placing the fronts of your ankles under the cushioned bar in front of you. You may need to adjust the chair so that your ankles sit comfortably underneath it. Slowly and gently push the cushioned bar up using your ankles and quadriceps. Then slowly and gently allow the bar to come down to its starting position. Take a deep breath and repeat this movement for the full amount of sets and reps.

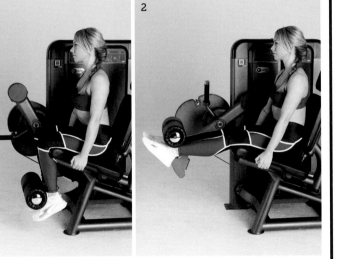

E 15 reps   **H** 12 reps

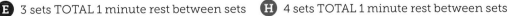

E 3 sets TOTAL 1 minute rest between sets   **H** 4 sets TOTAL 1 minute rest between sets

Monday + Thursday Lower Body

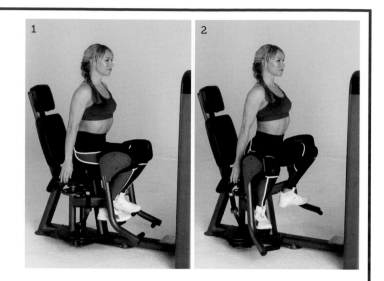

SUPERSET

1 Leg Abductor on Machine *Heavy weight*

Sit up straight on the machine and make sure the weight is right for you. Place your knees inside the pads. Keeping your back fully straight, push the pads outwards with your knees. This movement may seem like a leg movement, but this really should be (and feel like) a sitting thrust. The movement should be coming from your hips, into your glutes. Repeat this movement for the full amount of sets and reps.

E 15 reps   **H** 12 reps

2 Leg Adductor on Machine *Heavy weight*

Sit up straight on the machine and make sure the weight is right for you. Place your knees outside the pads. Keeping your back fully straight, push the pads inwards with your knees. This movement may seem like a leg movement, but this really should be (and feel like) an inner thigh exercise. Repeat this movement for the full amount of sets and reps.

E 15 reps   **H** 12 reps

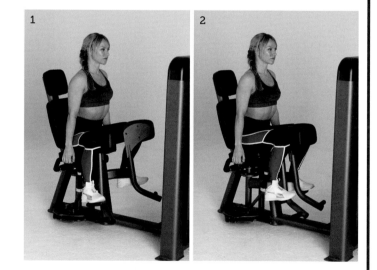

E 3 sets TOTAL 1 minute rest between sets   **H** 4 sets TOTAL 1 minute rest between sets

Tuesday + Friday Upper Body

 SUPERSET

1 Shoulder Press on Smith Machine
Heavy weight

Sit down and grab the handles with both hands. Push the handles up into the air and hold them there for a second before slowly bringing them back down. Repeat this movement for the full amount of sets and reps.

E 15 reps   **H** 12 reps

S 5 sets » 5 reps »
3 minutes rest between sets

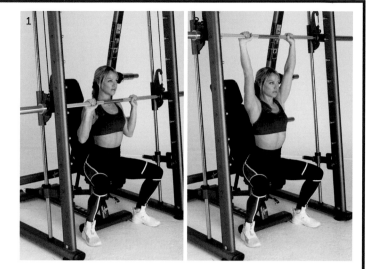

2 Walk Out Push-ups
Unweighted

Stand up straight with your feet hip-width apart. Allowing your knees to bend slightly, come down and forwards, so that your hands touch the floor, palms flat and shoulder-width apart. Crawl forwards until you are fully extended in a horizontal position. Keeping your back straight and bending only at the elbows, perform a push-up. Crawl your hands back until you can stand upright again. Repeat this movement to exhaust.

E To exhaust   **H** To exhaust

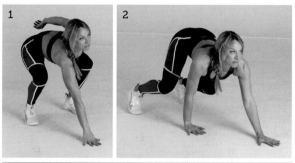

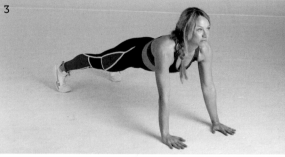

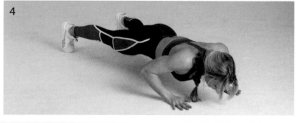

E 3 sets TOTAL 1 minute rest between sets

 4 sets TOTAL 1 minute rest between sets

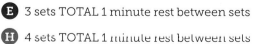

Tuesday + Friday Upper Body

 ★★ **SUPERSET**

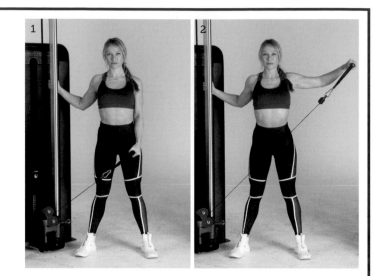

1 Lateral Raises on Cable Machine
Heavy weight

Attach the correct handle to the cable. With a slight bend in your elbow, and keeping your arm locked in this position, slowly raise the handle up into the air until your arm is horizontal. Allow the handle to slowly pull your arm back down into your starting position. Repeat this movement for the full amount of reps on each arm.

E 15 reps each arm

H 12 reps each arm

2 Front Raises on Cable Machine
Heavy weight

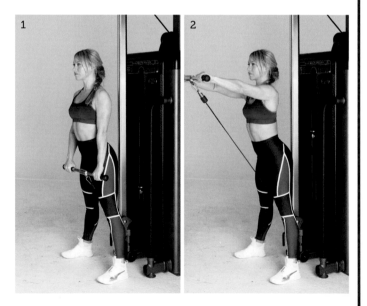

Attach the correct handle to the cable. With a slight bend in your elbows, and keeping your arms locked in this position, slowly raise the handle up into the air out in front of yourself. Allow the handle to slowly pull your arms back down into your starting position. Repeat this movement for the full amount of reps on each arm.

E 15 reps   **H** 12 reps

E 3 sets TOTAL 1 minute rest between sets   **H** 4 sets TOTAL 1 minute rest between sets

Bent Over Rows on Bench
Heavy dumbbell

Place a dumbbell on the floor on the right-hand side of a bench. Keeping your right foot on the ground and your toes pointing forwards, place your left knee in the centre of the bench, then bend over and grip the top of the bench with your left hand. Keeping your back straight, slowly pick up the dumbbell with your right hand, making sure to keep your arm in tight to your body as you do so. Pull the dumbbell up into your armpit region and hold the dumbbell there for a fraction of a second, then slowly bring it back down to extend your arm. Continue this movement for the full amount of sets and reps, then repeat with the other arm.

(E) 3 sets » 15 reps » 1 minute rest between sets

(H) 4 sets » 12 reps » 1 minute rest between sets

(S) 5 sets » 5 reps » 3 minutes rest between sets

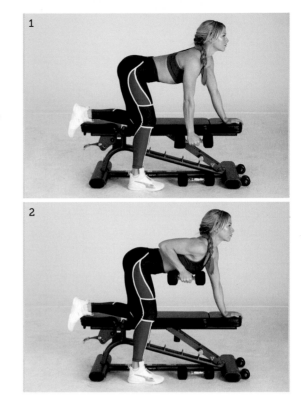

Rows are a great compound exercise that hit many of the muscles in your upper body and core. When performing rows, make sure you pull the weight into yourself with a swift, powerful movement, then lower it back down slowly and purposefully. You want to make sure the lift itself is powerful and the extension is slow and just as challenging.

Tuesday + Friday Upper Body

Chest Press with Olympic Bar
Heavy weight

(I would rather you use a bench press – a bench underneath a racked Olympic bar – for chest press exercies. However, if you have to use a Smith machine – illustrated here – that's fine.) Make sure the weight is the same each side – use clips if you need to. Lie back on the bench with your feet either side and flat against the floor. Reaching up, grip the bar with both your hands – your hands should be directly above your shoulders. Push the bar up so it is free from the holding, then bring it down slowly so it lightly touches your chest. Push the bar back up into the air and hold it there for a second before bringing it back down. Repeat this exercise for the full amount of sets and reps.

E 3 sets » 15 reps » 1 minute rest between sets

H 4 sets » 12 reps » 1 minute rest between sets

S 5 sets » 5 reps » 3 minutes rest between sets

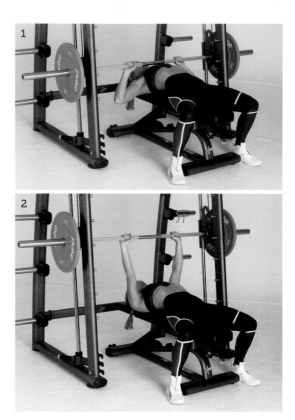

Bench press is another great exercise that will really challenge both your upper body and core. Take a deep breath in before you perform the push and exhale as you complete the movement. Breathing, and your timing of it, is pivotal to the strength and execution of every lift.

SUPERSET

1 Preacher Curls
Heavy weight

Load a weight you know you can lift on to the EZ bar (you may want to use clips) then straddle the bench. Lean forwards against the cushion, resting your chest against it and your armpits on top of it. Grab the bar with both hands, shoulder-width apart, using an underhand grip. Take a deep breath in and curl the EZ bar up to shoulder height. Slowly exhale as you allow the bar to creep back down towards its starting position. Take another deep breath and repeat the movement for the full amount of sets and reps.

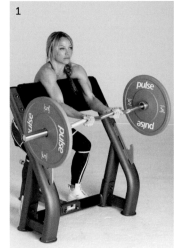
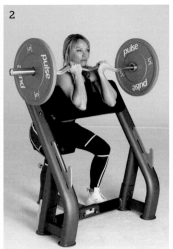

E 15 reps   **H** 12 reps

2 Tricep Rope Pulldowns
Heavy weight

Attach the rope pulley to the cable. Bring the cable up or down as necessary until it is shoulder height. Grip both sides of the rope with your hands. Stand upright and engage your core. Using your triceps, pull the rope down until your arms are fully extended (downwards). Simultaneously, pull both sides of the rope outwards, so they end up in front of your thighs. Hold this extension for a second, then slowly allow the rope to travel back up into your starting position. Take a breath and repeat this movement for the full amount of sets and reps.

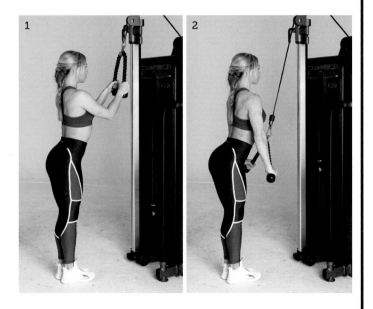

E 15 reps   **H** 12 reps

E 3 sets TOTAL 1 minute rest between sets   **H** 4 sets TOTAL 1 minute rest between sets

Wednesday + Saturday Back/Core

TRI SET

1 Wide Grip Pullups on Machine Assisted

Make sure the padded seat is upright. Facing the machine, grip the bars that are furthest apart using an overhand grip and place your knees on top of the seat. Slowly allow your body to drop down underneath the bars. Once your arms are fully extended, slowly pull yourself back up into a wide-grip pull-up position. Hold this for a second before allowing yourself to come back down to your starting position. Take a deep breath and repeat this movement for the full amount of sets and reps.

E 15 reps   **H** 12 reps

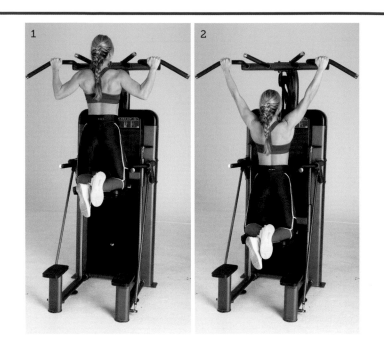

2 Close Grip Pullups on Machine Assisted

Make sure the padded seat is upright. Facing the machine, grip the bars above you that are closest together using an underhand grip. Place your knees on top of the seat, then slowly allow your body to drop down underneath the bars. Once your arms are fully extended, slowly pull yourself back up into a pull-up position. Hold this position for a second before allowing yourself to come back down again. Take a deep breath and repeat this movement for the full amount of sets and reps.

E 15 reps   **H** 12 reps

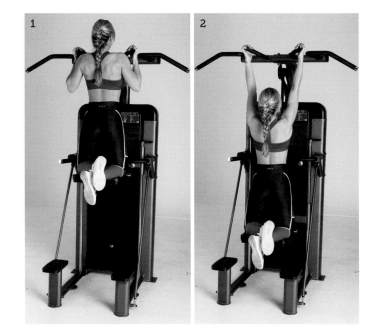

3 Tricep Dips on Machine Assisted

Make sure the padded seat is upright and the bars on either side of the machine are as close together as possible (they are often adjustable). Grip the bars and place your knees on top of the padded seat. Keeping your elbows in tight to your sides, slowly allow your body to drop down. When you have come down as far as possible, slowly push yourself back up, using your triceps. Take a deep breath and repeat this movement for the full amount of sets and reps.

E 15 reps   **H** 12 reps

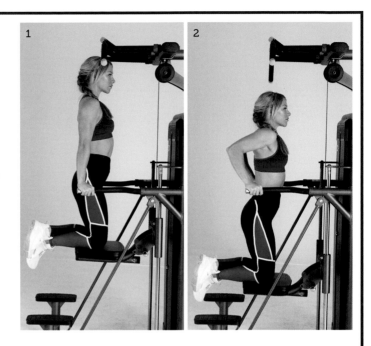

E 3 sets TOTAL 1 minute rest between sets   **H** 4 sets TOTAL 1 minute rest between sets

If your gym doesn't have an Assisted Machine, simply tie a resistance band around a high bar and rest your feet (or bended knees) on the inside of it. This way, when you go to perform the pull, you are assisted in the movement by the band itself.

Wednesday + Saturday Back/Core

SUPERSET

1 Wide Grip Rows on Machine Heavy weight

You can do these on a static machine or using the cable machine (as illustrated), depending on what equipment your gym has. Either sit with your legs either side of the machine or stand with your feet together and knees bent. Holding the bar using an overhand grip, take a deep breath and slowly and gently pull the bar into your chest. Hold it against yourself for a second, then slowly and gently let it pull you back to the starting position. Take a deep breath and repeat this movement for the full amount of sets and reps.

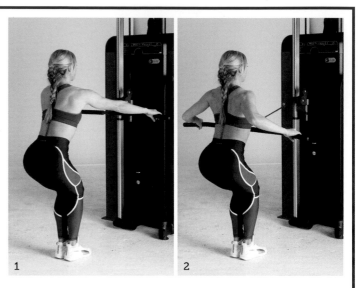

E 15 reps **H** 12 reps

2 Close Grip Rows on Machine Heavy weight

You can do these on a static machine (as illustrated) or using the cable machine, depending on what equipment your gym has. Sit down with your legs either side of the machine and grip the handles in front of you with an inverted grip. Take a deep breath and, slowly and gently, pull the handles into your chest. Hold the handles against yourself for a second, then slowly and gently let them pull you back to the starting position. Take a deep breath and repeat this movement for the full amount of sets and reps.

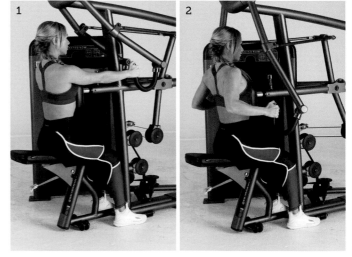

E 15 reps **H** 12 reps

E 3 sets TOTAL 1 minute rest between sets   **H** 4 sets TOTAL 1 minute rest between sets

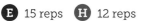

SUPERSET

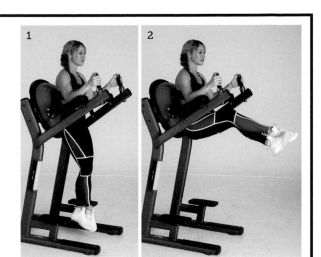

1
2

Leg Raises on Machine
Unweighted

Stand on the machine. Keep your back straight against the back pad and grip both the handles. Let your legs dangle underneath you and cross your ankles. Slowly raise your legs up in front of you, then slowly allow them to come back down to your starting position. Repeat this movement fluidly to exhaust.

E 1 set to exhaust

H 1 set to exhaust

The Plank Unweighted

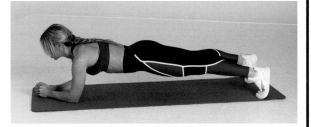

You may need a mat or cushion for your elbows during this exercise. Lie on your front with your feet hip-width apart. Rest on your elbows and keep your forearms flat against the mat. Make sure your elbows are underneath your shoulders. Pushing against your toes and forearms, raise your body up into an elevated plank. Do not allow your spine to curve, either concavely or convexly – you want a straight back. Hold this position to exhaust. If you are struggling, feel free to transfer your weight from one foot to another, essentially shuffling your feet while holding the plank position.

E 1 set to exhaust

H 1 set to exhaust

SUNDAY = FULL REST DAY

Week 3 Overload Focused
(increased weight / volume / intensity)

Monday + Thursday = Lower Body

Tuesday + Friday = Upper Body

Wednesday + Saturday = Back/Core

Sunday = Rest day

You'll see this is a 6-day weight-lifting plan. However, you only need to train for 4 or 5 days a week, if you'd prefer.

As long as you make sure you train your body evenly – at least 1 day on your Lower Body, 1 day on your Upper Body and 1 day on your Back/Core – feel free to weight-train anywhere between 4 and 6 days a week, taking rest days as and when you need them.

Key to symbols

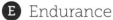 Endurance

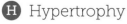 Hypertrophy

S Strength. If Strength is your goal but the symbol is missing from an exercise, leave the exercise out.

Monday + Thursday Lower Body

Squats on Squat Rack with Olympic Bar Heavy weight

Make sure the weight is the same each side – use clips if you need to. Find the centre of the horizontal bar and duck underneath it, so the bar is resting across your shoulders. Take hold of the bar either side of your shoulders and come up slightly on your tiptoes. Remove the bar from its holdings and take a few cautious steps backwards. Place your feet hip-width apart, or slightly further if that is a more comfortable squat position for you, and make sure your toes are either pointing forwards or slightly outwards, whichever is more comfortable. Standing up straight and bending only at the hip and knees, come down into a low squat before pushing back up through your heels to a standing position, squeezing your glutes as you do so. Take a breath and repeat this movement for the full amount of sets and reps.

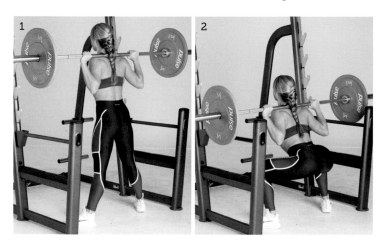

E 3 sets » 15 reps »
1 minute rest between sets

H 4 sets » 12 reps »
1 minute rest between sets

S **INCREASE WEIGHT**
3 sets » 3 rep »
3 minutes rest between sets

Deadlift with Olympic Bar
Heavy weight

Make sure the weight is the same each side – use clips if you need to. Place the bar in front of your feet. Stand up straight with your feet hip-width apart, toes pointing forwards. Keeping your back straight and bending only at the hips and knees, crouch down so your hands are able to reach the bar. Grasp the bar either side of your legs, placing one hand in an overhand grip and the other in an underhand grip (whichever is more comfortable). Once you have a good grip, stand up straight, pushing down through your heels as you do so. As you come into a fully vertical standing position, squeeze your buttocks at the top of the movement. Keeping the bar against your legs, slowly allow it to pull you back down to the ground again, keeping your back straight and bending only at the hips and knees at all times. Allow the bar to hit the floor, take a breath and repeat the lift for the full amount of sets and reps.

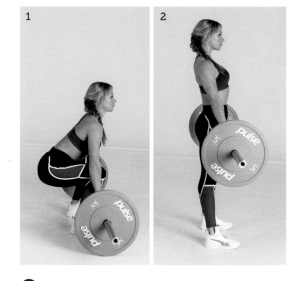

E 3 sets » 15 reps » 1 minute rest between sets

H 4 sets » 12 reps » 1 minute rest between sets

S **INCREASE WEIGHT**
3 sets » 3 reps » 3 minutes rest between sets

WEEK 3

Monday + Thursday Lower Body

Hip Thrusts on Smith Machine Heavy weight

(Please note: the illustration shows the Smith unweighted – this exercise should be weighted.)
Place a bench about 0.5m behind you, so you are sandwiched between the Smith and the bench.
Lower the bar so it is about 30cm off the ground. Sit down between the bar and the bench, facing
the bar and resting your upper back and shoulder blades on the edge of the bench. Place a bar pad
(a black, cushioned tube) around the centre of the horizontal bar. Place your feet hip-width apart
and keep your toes pointing forwards or slightly outwards. Place your hips underneath the bar and
your hands either side of your hips. Unhook the bar from the machine – keep it unhooked using
your grip – and thrust up into the air, through your glutes, squeezing them tight at the top of the
movement. Hold this position for a few seconds before coming back down until your buttocks are
just above the ground. Take a breath and repeat this movement for the full amount of sets and reps.

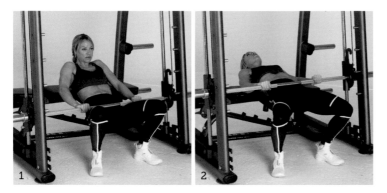

E 3 sets » 15 reps »
1 minute rest between sets

H 4 sets » 12 reps »
1 minute rest between sets

Walking Weighted Lunges Heavy barbell

With the barbell lying across the back of your shoulders, stand up straight and take a big step forward,
coming down into a deep lunge. Remember to keep your back upright and your lunged knee directly
above your toes at all times. Push yourself back into a standing position and repeat this move with
the opposite leg. Repeat these steps for the full amount of sets and reps.

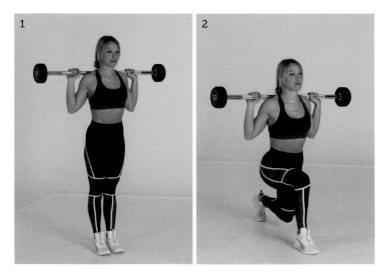

E 3 sets » 15 steps each leg »
1 minute rest between sets

H 4 sets » 12 steps each leg »
1 minute rest between sets

SUPERSET

1 Leg Curl Machine
Heavy weight

Sit down on the machine, placing the backs of your ankles over the cushioned bar in front of you. You may need to adjust the chair so that your ankles sit comfortably on top of it. Slowly and gently push the cushioned bar down using your ankles and hamstrings. Then slowly and gently allow the bar to come back up to its starting position. Take a deep breath and repeat this movement for the full amount of sets and reps.

E 15 reps **H** 12 reps

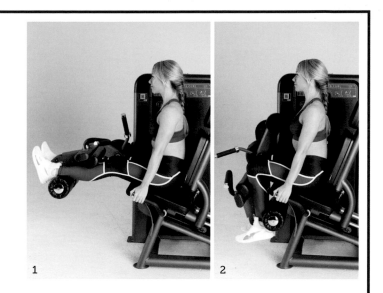

2 Leg Extension Machine Heavy weight

Sit down on the machine, placing the fronts of your ankles under the cushioned bar in front of you. You may need to adjust the chair so that your ankles sit comfortably underneath it. Slowly and gently push the cushioned bar up using your ankles and quadriceps. Then slowly and gently allow the bar to come down to its starting position. Take a deep breath and repeat this movement for the full amount of sets and reps.

E 15 reps **H** 12 reps

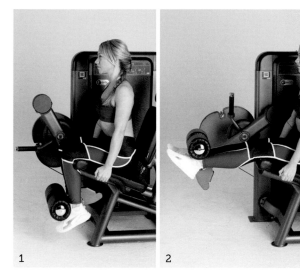

E 3 sets TOTAL 1 minute rest between sets   **H** 4 sets TOTAL 1 minute rest between sets

Tuesday + Friday Upper Body

Chest Press with Olympic Bar
Heavy weight

(I would rather you use a bench press – a bench underneath a racked Olympic bar – for chest press exercises. However, if you have to use a Smith machine – illustrated here – that's fine.) Make sure the weight is the same each side – use clips if you need to. Lie back on the bench with your feet either side and flat on the floor. Reaching up, grip the bar with both your hands – your hands should be directly above your shoulders. Push the bar up so it is free from the holding, then bring it down slowly so it lightly touches your chest. Push the bar back up into the air and hold it there for a second before bringing it back down. Repeat this movement for the full amount of sets and reps.

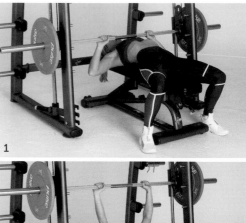
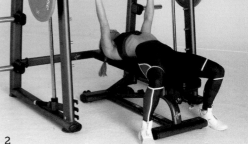

E 3 sets » 15 reps » 1 minute rest between sets

H 4 sets » 12 reps » 1 minute rest between sets

S INCREASE WEIGHT
3 sets » 3 reps » 3 minutes rest between sets

Seated Smith Press
Heavy weight

Place a bench underneath the Smith and make sure the seat is upright. The weight should be one that will challenge you. Sit upright with the bar directly in front of your chest. Grip the bar with both hands, making sure your hands are shoulder-width apart. Push the bar up into the air above your head, then slowly allow the bar to come back down to chest height. Repeat this movement for the full amount of sets and reps.

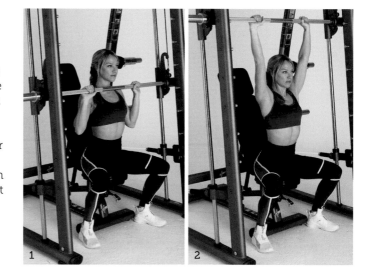

E 3 sets » 15 reps »
1 minute rest between sets

H 4 sets » 12 reps »
1 minute rest between sets

S INCREASE WEIGHT
3 sets » 3 reps »
3 minutes rest between sets

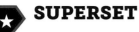 **SUPERSET**

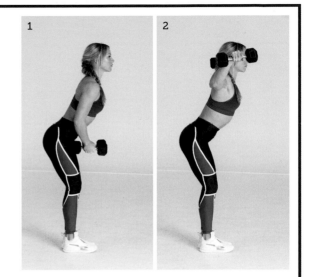

1 Lateral Raise Hold with Dumbbells Heavy weight

Make sure the weight is the same in each hand. Stand up straight with your knees slightly bent and your feet together. Grip the dumbbells in front of your crotch, lightly touching each other. Lean ever-so-slightly forward with your upper body, keeping an ever-so-slight arch in your lower back. Keeping a slight bend in your elbows and bowing them outwards slightly, slowly and gradually raise the dumbbells out either side of you, until your arms are horizontal, like an eagle in flight. Hold this position to exhaust.

E Hold to exhaust   **H** Hold to exhaust

2 Front Raise Hold with Dumbbells Heavy weight

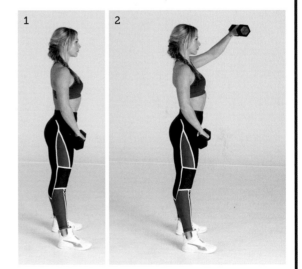

Make sure the weight is the same in each hand. Stand up straight with your feet hip-width apart and your toes pointing forwards. Grip the dumbbells horizontally, using an overhand grip, and allow them to hang together in front of your crotch. Keeping your back straight at all times, take a deep breath and slowly raise one dumbbell. Keep a slight bend in your elbow as you do so. Hold this position to exhaust. Repeat with the other arm.

E Hold to exhaust   **H** Hold to exhaust

E 3 sets TOTAL 1 minute rest between sets   **H** 4 sets TOTAL 1 minute rest between sets

Tuesday + Friday Upper Body

★★ SUPERSET

1 Close Grip Pullups on Machine Assisted

Make sure the padded seat is upright. Grip the bars above you that are closest together using an underhand grip. Place your knees on top of the padded seat, then slowly allow your body to drop down underneath the bars. Once your arms are fully extended, slowly pull yourself back up into a pull-up position. Hold this position for a second before allowing yourself to come back down again. Take a deep breath and repeat this movement for the full amount of sets and reps.

OR Unassisted

Grip the bars that are closest together using an underhand grip. Allow your body to drop down underneath the bars then swiftly pull yourself back up again. Take a deep breath and repeat this movement for the full amount of sets and reps.

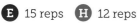

E 15 reps **H** 12 reps

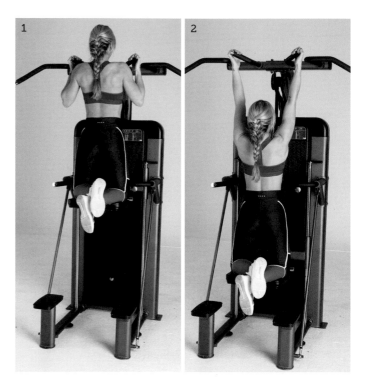

I would like you to try and complete these sets and reps unassisted. However, if you are not quite there yet, just make sure you lower the assistance and continue to get stronger in the lift.

2 Tricep Dips on Machine Assisted

Make sure the padded seat is upright and the bars on either side of the machine are as close together as possible (they are often adjustable). Grip the bars and place your knees on top of the padded seat. Keeping your elbows in tight to your sides, slowly allow your body to drop down. When you have come down as far as possible, slowly push yourself back up, using your triceps. Take a deep breath and repeat this movement for the full amount of sets and reps.

OR Unassisted

Grip the bars. Keeping your elbows in tight to your sides, slowly allow your body to drop down. When you have come down as far as possible, slowly push yourself back up, using your triceps. Take a deep breath and repeat this movement for the full amount of sets and reps.

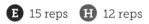 15 reps   **H** 12 reps

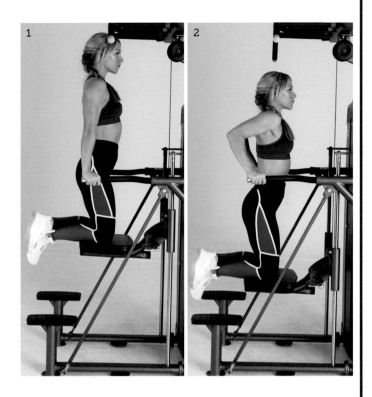

E 3 sets TOTAL 1 minute rest between sets   **H** 4 sets TOTAL 1 minute rest between sets

Wednesday + Saturday Back/Core

★★ SUPERSET

1 Wide Grip Pulldowns on Machine Heavy weight

You can do this on a specific cable machine with a bench attached, or you can improvise as I have done in the illustration, by pulling a bench up close to any cable machine. Attach the long bar to the cable machine and make sure it's at its highest setting. Sit down on the bench, fully upright, and grab the bar on either side of the cable with an overhand grip. Pull the bar down in front of your chest and slowly let it pull your arms back up again. Repeat this movement for the full amount of sets and reps.

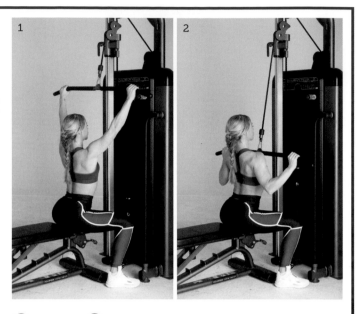

E 15 reps   **H** 12 reps

2 Close Grip Pulldowns on Machine Heavy weight

You can do this on a specific cable machine with a bench attached, or you can improvise, as I have done in the illustration, by pulling a bench up close to any cable machine. Attach any bar to the cable machine and make sure it's at its highest setting. Sit down on the bench, fully upright, and grab the bar on either side of the cable with an underhand grip. Pull the bar down in front of your chest and slowly let it pull your arms back up again. Repeat this movement for the full amount of sets and reps.

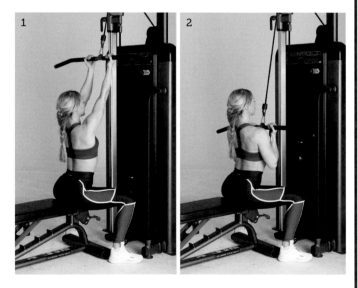

E 15 reps   **H** 12 reps

E 3 sets TOTAL 1 minute rest between sets   **H** 4 sets TOTAL 1 minute rest between sets

Hyperextensions on Machine
Heavy weight

(Please note that the illustration shows an unweighted hyperextension on the mat. If your gym has a hyperextension machine, though, this is preferable. Hold a weight plate against your chest as you do the hyperextensions on the machine.) Slowly bow your body back into a lower back crunch (another name for this exercise is a reverse sit up). Make sure you engage your glutes and core while doing this exercise. Hold this position for a few seconds then repeat the movement for the full amount of sets and reps.

E 3 sets » 15 reps » 1 minute rest between sets

H 4 sets » 12 reps » 1 minute rest between sets

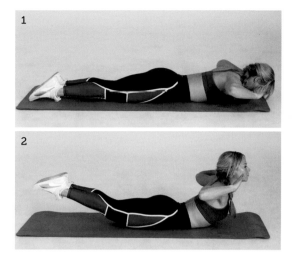

You will feel pulldowns working your entire upper body and core. They are a great compound movement that will hugely benefit your overall strength and muscle development. Even though these pulls are not traditional in a strength training / powerlifting programme, they can be great accessory work for this goal, too!

Wednesday + Saturday Back/Core

Bent Over Rows on Bench
Heavy dumbbell

Place a dumbbell on the floor on the right-hand side of a bench. Keeping your right foot on the ground and your toes pointing forwards, place your left knee in the centre of the bench, then bend over and grip the top of the bench with your left hand. Keeping your back straight, slowly pick up the dumbbell with your right hand, making sure to keep your arm in tight to your body as you do so. Pull the dumbbell up into your armpit region and hold the dumbbell there for a fraction of a second, then slowly bring it back down to extend your arm. Continue this movement for the full amount of sets and reps, then repeat with the other arm.

E 3 sets » 15 reps » 1 minute rest between sets

H 4 sets » 12 reps » 1 minute rest between sets

S 3 sets » 3 reps » 3 minutes rest between sets

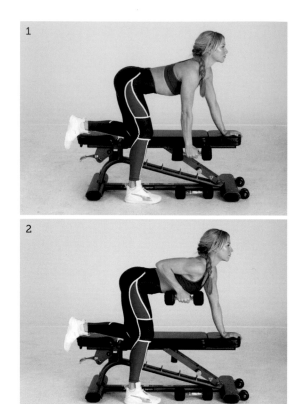

Whether you do bent over rows with a dumbbell or a barbell is up to you. Both will challenge and hit the intended muscle, albeit in slightly different ways. It's always good to switch up the specifics of exercises in order to keep challenging our lifting and hitting different areas of muscle.

Kettlebell Swings Heavy kettlebell

Stand over the kettlebell, feet slightly wider than hip-width apart. Squat down and grip the kettlebell with both hands. Pull your shoulders back, engage your core and thrust through your glutes and hips, launching the kettlebell up into the air in front of you. Aim to swing up to chest height, then allow the kettlebell to swing back down between your legs, keeping full control of your upper body while this happens. Repeat this movement fluidly and aggressively for the full amount of sets and reps.

E 3 sets » 15 reps » 1 minute rest between sets   **H** 4 sets » 12 reps » 1 minute rest between sets

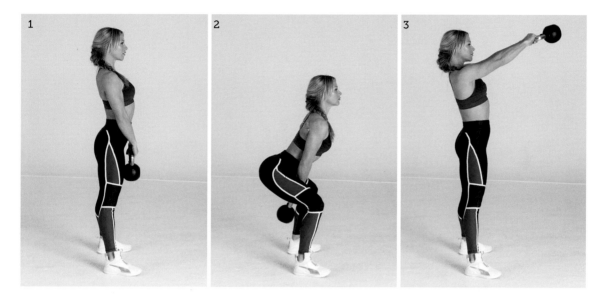

The Plank Unweighted on mat

You may need a mat or cushion for your elbows during this exercise. Lie on your front with your feet hip-width apart. Rest on your elbows and keep your forearms flat against the mat. Make sure your elbows are below your shoulders. Pushing against your toes and forearms, raise your body up into an elevated plank. Do not allow your spine to curve, either concavely or convexly – you want a straight back. Hold this position to exhaust. If you are struggling, feel free to transfer your weight from one foot to another, essentially shuffling your feet while holding the plank position.

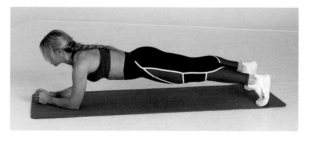

E 1 set to exhaust   **H** 1 set to exhaust

SUNDAY = FULL REST DAY

Advanced

Week 4 Overload Focused
(increased weight / volume / intensity)

Monday + Thursday = Lower Body

Tuesday + Friday = Upper Body

Wednesday + Saturday = Back/Core

Sunday = Rest day

You'll see this is a 6-day weight-lifting plan. However, you only need to train for 4 or 5 days a week, if you'd prefer.

As long as you make sure you train your body evenly – at least 1 day on your Lower Body, 1 day on your Upper Body and 1 day on your Back/Core – feel free to weight-train anywhere between 4 and 6 days a week, taking rest days as and when you need them.

Key to symbols

E Endurance

H Hypertrophy

S Strength. If Strength is your goal but the symbol is missing from an exercise, leave the exercise out.

Monday + Thursday Lower Body

Squats on Squat Rack with Olympic Bar Heavy weight

Make sure the weight is the same each side – use clips if you need to. Find the centre of the horizontal bar and duck underneath it, so the bar is resting across your shoulders. Take hold of the bar either side of your shoulders and come up slightly on your tiptoes. Remove the bar from its holdings and take a few cautious steps backwards. Place your feet hip-width apart, or slightly further if that is a more comfortable squat position for you, and make sure your toes are either pointing forwards or slightly outwards, whichever is more comfortable. Standing up straight and bending only at the hip and knees, come down into a low squat before pushing back up through your heels to a standing position, squeezing your glutes as you do so. Take a breath and repeat this movement for the full amount of sets and reps.

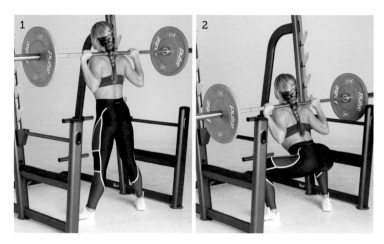

E 3 sets » 15 reps »
1 minute rest between sets

H 4 sets » 12 reps »
1 minute rest between sets

S Work to your 1RPM
(1 rep max weight)

Front Squats on Smith Machine Heavy weight

Make sure the weight is the same on each side of the bar. Find the centre of the horizontal bar and grip it with both of your hands. Place your feet hip-width apart, or slightly further if that is a more comfortable squat position for you, and make sure your toes are either pointing forwards or slightly outwards, whichever is more comfortable. Standing close to the bar so it is pressing into your chest and the fronts of your shoulders, unhook the bar from the machine – keep it unhooked using your grip. Standing up straight and bending only at the hip and knees, come down into a low squat before pushing back up through your heels to a standing position, squeezing your glutes as you do so. Take a breath and repeat this movement for the full amount of sets and reps.

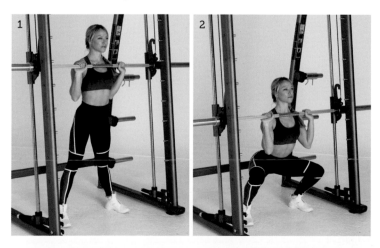

E 3 sets » 15 reps »
1 minute rest between sets

H 4 sets » 12 reps »
1 minute rest between sets

Monday + Thursday Lower Body

Hyperextensions on Machine
Heavy weight

(Please note that the illustration shows an unweighted hyperextension on the mat. If your gym has a hyperextension machine, though, this is preferable. Hold a weight plate against your chest as you do the hyperextensions on the machine.) Sowly bow your body back into a lower back crunch (another name for this exercise is a reverse sit up). Make sure you engage your glutes and core while doing this exercise. Hold this position for a few seconds then repeat this movement for the full amount of sets and reps.

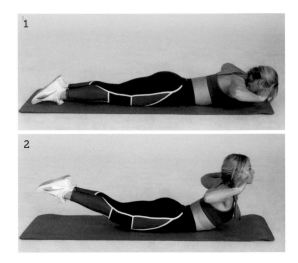

E 3 sets » 15 reps » 1 minute rest between sets

H 4 sets » 12 reps » 1 minute rest between sets

Deadlift with Olympic Bar
Heavy weight

Make sure the weight is the same each side – use clips if you need to. Place the bar in front of your feet. Stand up straight with your feet hip-width apart, toes pointing forwards. Keeping your back straight and bending only at the hips and knees, crouch down so your hands are able to reach the bar. Grasp the bar either side of your legs, placing one hand in an overhand grip and the other in an underhand grip (whichever is more comfortable is fine). Once you have a good grip, stand up straight, pushing down through your heels as you do so. As you come into a fully vertical standing position, squeeze your buttocks at the top of the movement. Keeping the bar against your legs, slowly allow it to pull you back down to the ground again, keeping your back straight and bending only at the hips and knees at all times. Allow the bar to hit the floor, take a breath and repeat the lift for the full amount of sets and reps.

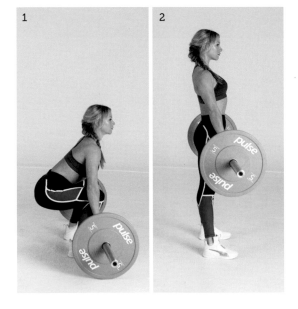

E 3 sets » 15 reps » 1 minute rest between sets

H 4 sets » 12 reps » 1 minute rest between sets

S Work to your 1RPM (1 rep max)

Donkey Kick Backs on Smith Machine OR Cable Machine
Heavy weight

Place a thick mat directly underneath the Smith bar. Make sure the weight is the same on each side of the bar. Kneel on the mat slightly in front of the bar and get down on all fours. Place the ball of your right foot under the bar and push up a little, then roll the bar back a little using the ball of your foot, and it will unhook itself. This needs a little skill and it may take a few sessions until you can do it seamlessly, but you will get there. Slowly and gently bring your knee down towards the mat and then push up until your leg is almost fully extended, always keeping a slight bend in the knee. Take a breath and repeat this movement for the full amount of sets and reps on each leg.

OR You can also do DKBs on the cable machine. Attach a Velcro ankle strap to the cable, stand upright and kick your leg back into the air while engaging your glute.

(E) 3 sets » 15 reps » 1 minute rest between sets

(H) 4 sets » 12 reps » 1 minute rest between sets

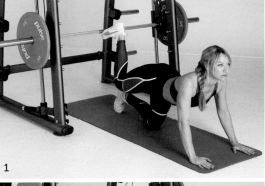

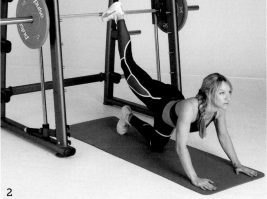

Leg Press on Machine
Heavy weight

Sit down and place your feet hip-width apart on the plate in front of you (or slightly further apart if that is more comfortable). Point your toes upwards, or slightly outwards. Pushing through the flats of your feet, slowly and gently push against the plate. Depending on the machine, the force will either push the plate away from your seat, or your seat away from the plate. When you have fully extended (without locking your knees out – you should always keep a slight bend in them when performing a lower body lift), slowly come back into your starting position. Take a breath and repeat this movement for the full amount of sets and reps. Finish with light calf presses to exhaust.

(E) 3 sets » 15 reps » 1 minute rest between sets

(H) 4 sets » 12 reps » 1 minute rest between sets

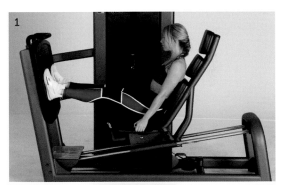

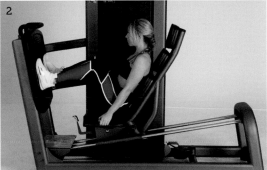

Tuesday + Friday Upper Body

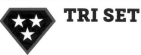 **TRI SET**

1 Seated Dumbbell Press
Heavy dumbbells

Adjust the bench so it's upright then sit up straight on the bench with your back against it. Hold a dumbbell in each hand and rest them on top of your thighs if need be. Bring them up to shoulder height and hold them horizontally. Push both dumbbells up into the air and gently touch them together at the top of the movement. Slowly bring them back down to shoulder height and repeat this movement for the full sets and reps.

E 15 rep   **H** 12 reps

S Work to your 1 RPM (1 rep max)

Please note: You will need someone to spot you if you press dumbbells to your 1 RPM. Alternatively, you could do a Smith press instead.

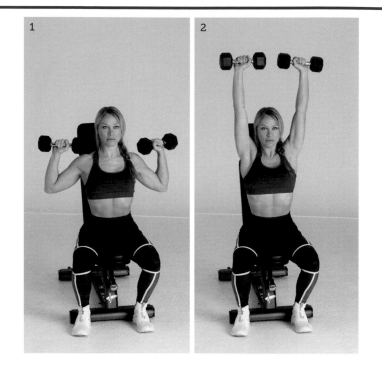

If you are strength training and trying to hit your 1 RPM, I suggest you ask an experienced lifter, PT or gym instructor to spot you.

2 Lateral Raises
Heavy dumbbells

Make sure the weight is the same in each hand. Stand up straight with your knees slightly bent, your feet together. Grip the dumbbells in front of your crotch, lightly touching each other. Lean ever-so-slightly forward with your upper body, keeping a slight arch in your lower back. Keeping a slight bend in your elbows and bowing them outwards slightly, slowly and gradually raise the dumbbells out either side of you, until your arms are horizontal, like an eagle in flight. Hold this position for a fraction of a second, then slowly bring your arms back down to your starting position. Take a breath and repeat this movement for the full amount of sets and reps.

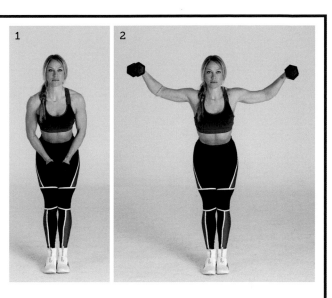

E 15 reps   **H** 12 reps

3 Front Raises Heavy dumbbells

Make sure the weight is the same in each hand. Stand up straight with your feet hip-width apart and your toes pointing forwards. Grip the dumbbells horizontally, using an overhand grip, and allow them to hang together in front of your crotch. Keeping your back straight at all times, take a deep breath and slowly raise one of the dumbbells. Keep a slight bend in your elbow as you do so. Hold the dumbbell in its raised position for a fraction of a second, then slowly bring it back down. Repeat with the other arm. Continue this movement alternately for the full amount of sets and reps.

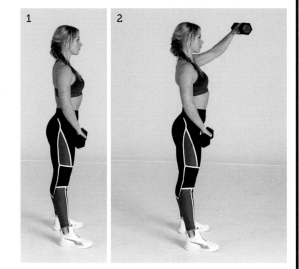

E 15 reps   **H** 12 reps

E 3 sets TOTAL 1 minute rest between sets   **H** 4 sets TOTAL 1 minute rest between sets

Tuesday + Friday Upper Body

Bent Over Rows with Olympic Bar Heavy weight

Stand up straight with your feet hip-width apart. Grab the bar with both hands and pull your shoulders back. Keeping an arch in your back and holding the bar against your lower body, slowly come down into a hamstring stretch until you have reached your full range of motion. Once there, pull the bar up into your ribcage, then slowly lower it back down again. Take a deep breath and repeat this movement for the full amount of sets and reps.

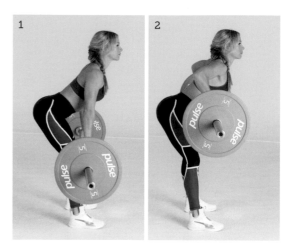

E 3 sets » 15 reps » 1 minute rest between sets

H 4 sets » 12 reps » 1 minute rest between sets

S Work to your 1 RPM (1 rep max)

Chest Press with Olympic Bar
Heavy weight

(I would rather you use a bench press – a bench underneath a racked Olympic bar – for chest press exercies. However, if you have to use a Smith machine – illustrated here – that's fine.) Make sure the weight is the same each side – use clips if you need to. Lie back on the bench with your feet either side and flat on the floor. Reaching up, grip the bar with both your hands – your hands should be directly above your shoulders. Push the bar up so it is free from the holding, then bring it down slowly so it lightly touches your chest. Push the bar back up into the air and hold it there for a second before bringing it back down. Repeat this movement for the full amount of sets and reps.

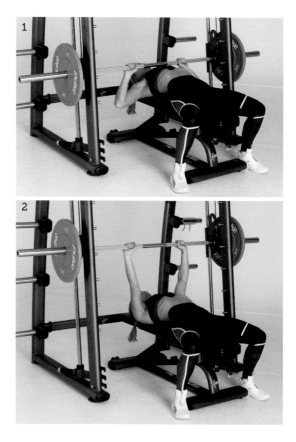

E 3 sets » 15 reps » 1 minute rest between sets

H 4 sets » 12 reps » 1 minute rest between sets

S Work to your 1 RPM (1 rep max)

Chest Fly on Bench
Heavy dumbbells

Make sure the weight is the same in each hand. Sit on the bench with your feet flat on the floor on either side and grip the dumbbells in your hands, resting them on top of your thighs. Lie down on the bench. Keeping the dumbbells vertical in your grip, extend your arms out either side of your body at chest height. Then, as if you are hugging a beach ball, and keeping a slight bend in your elbows, bring the dumbbells together above your body. Slowly bring the dumbbells back down to the starting position. Take a breath and repeat this move for the full amount of sets and reps.

E 3 sets » 15 reps »
1 minute rest between sets

H 4 sets » 12 reps »
1 minute rest between sets

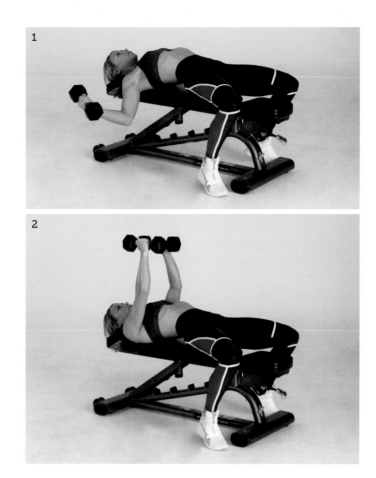

Feel free to switch up your bench press to an incline or decline bench, in order to hit different areas of your chest and continue to challenge and push yourself in the lift. This will also hugely benefit your aesthetic results.

Wednesday + Saturday Back/Core

Kettlebell Swings
Heavy kettlebell

Stand over the kettlebell, feet slightly wider than hip-width apart. Squat down and grip the kettlebell with both hands. Pull your shoulders back, engage your core and thrust through your glutes and hips, launching the kettlebell up into the air in front of you. Aim to swing up to chest height, then allow the kettlebell to swing back down between your legs, keeping full control of your upper body while this happens. Repeat this movement fluidly and aggressively for the full amount of sets and reps.

E 3 sets » 15 reps » 1 minute rest between sets

H 4 sets » 12 reps » 1 minute rest between sets

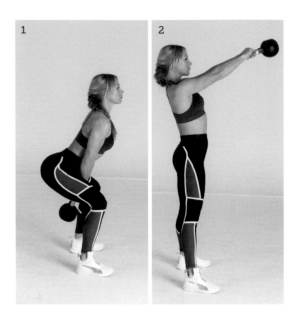

Dumbbell Pullovers
Heavy dumbbells

Sit on the bench, legs either side of it, and grip the dumbbell (vertically) between your legs. Lie down and, as you do so, raise the dumbbell up in the air, directly above your face. Now adjust your grip by opening your hands, allowing the weight of the dumbbell to rest against the flats of your palms, gripping around its base with your fingers. Allow the dumbbell to slowly and gently come behind you, so that it is behind your head and behind the bench. Slowly and gently bring it back up into the air, above your face, into your starting position. Take a deep breath and repeat this movement for the full amount of sets and reps.

E 3 sets » 15 reps » 1 minute rest between sets

H 4 sets » 12 reps » 1 minute rest between sets

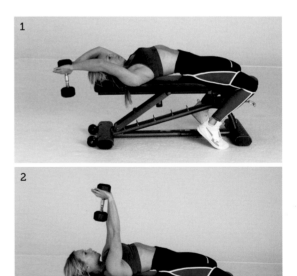

SUPERSET

1 Single Arm Wide Grip Rows
Heavy weight

Sit down with your legs either side of the machine and grip the handle in front of you with an inverted grip. Take a deep breath, then slowly and gently pull the handle in to your chest. Hold the handle against you for a second, then slowly and gently let it pull you back to the starting position. Take a deep breath and repeat this movement for the full amount of sets and reps.

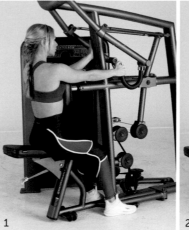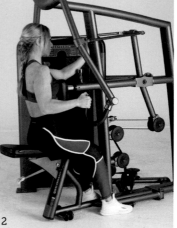

E 15 reps   **H** 12 reps

2 Single Arm Close Grip Rows
Heavy weight

You can do these sitting on the floor in front of the cable machine or standing, whichever you prefer. I like to do the exercises standing when I can, as per the illustration. Grip one handle with an inverted grip, take a deep breath then slowly and gently pull the handle into your chest. Hold the handle against yourself for a second, then slowly and gently let it pull you back to the starting position. Take a deep breath and repeat this movement for the full amount of reps, on each arm.

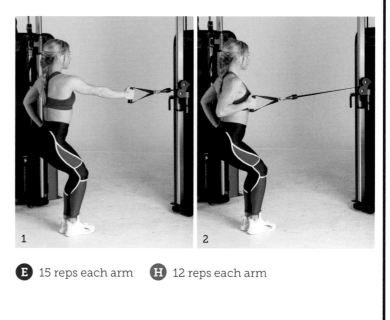

E 15 reps each arm   **H** 12 reps each arm

E 3 sets TOTAL 1 minute rest between sets   **H** 4 sets TOTAL 1 minute rest between sets

Wednesday + Saturday Back/Core

Wide Grip Pullups on Machine Assisted

Make sure the padded seat is upright on the machine. Grip the bars that are furthest apart using an overhand grip and place your knees on top of the padded seat. Slowly allow your body to drop down underneath the bars. Once your arms are fully extended, slowly pull yourself back up into a wide-grip pull-up position. Hold this for a second before allowing yourself to come back down to your starting position. Take a deep breath and repeat this movement for the full amount of sets and reps.

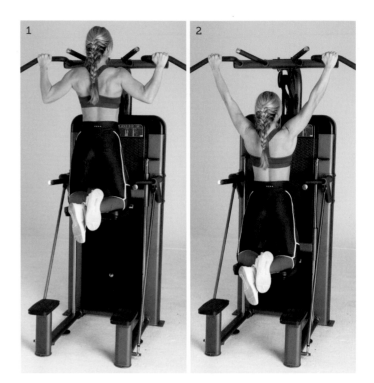

E 3 sets » 15 reps » 1 minute rest between sets

H 4 sets » 12 reps » 1 minute rest between sets

OR Unassisted

Grip the bars that are furthest apart in an overhand grip. Slowly allow your body to drop down underneath the bars and then swiftly pull yourself back up. Take a deep breath and repeat this movement for the full amount of sets and reps.

E 3 sets to exhaust » 1 minute rest between sets

H 4 sets to exhaust » 1 minute rest between sets

Remember – I can't tell you how strong you are, only you know how you feel. Just make sure you consciously and consistently push yourself in every session and with every lift.

Close Grip Pullups on Machine Assisted

Make sure the padded seat is upright, ready for you to kneel on. Grip the bars above you that are closest together using an underhand grip. Place your knees on top of the padded seat, then slowly allow your body to drop down underneath the bars. Once your arms are fully extended, slowly pull yourself back up into a pull-up position. Hold this position for a second before allowing yourself to come back down again. Take a deep breath and repeat this movement for the full amount of sets and reps.

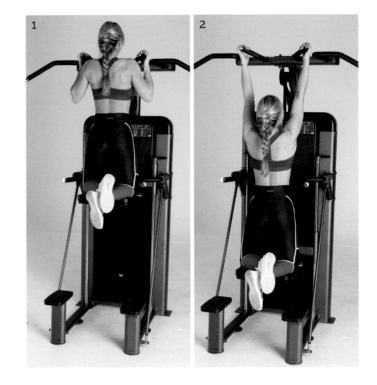

E 3 sets » 15 reps »
1 minute rest between sets

H 4 sets » 12 reps »
1 minute rest between sets

OR Unassisted

Grip the bars that are closest together in an underhand grip. Slowly allow your body to drop down underneath the bars then swiftly pull yourself back up again. Take a deep breath and repeat this movement for the full amount of sets and reps.

E 3 sets to exhaust »
1 minute rest between sets

H 4 sets to exhaust »
1 minute rest between sets

SUNDAY = FULL REST DAY

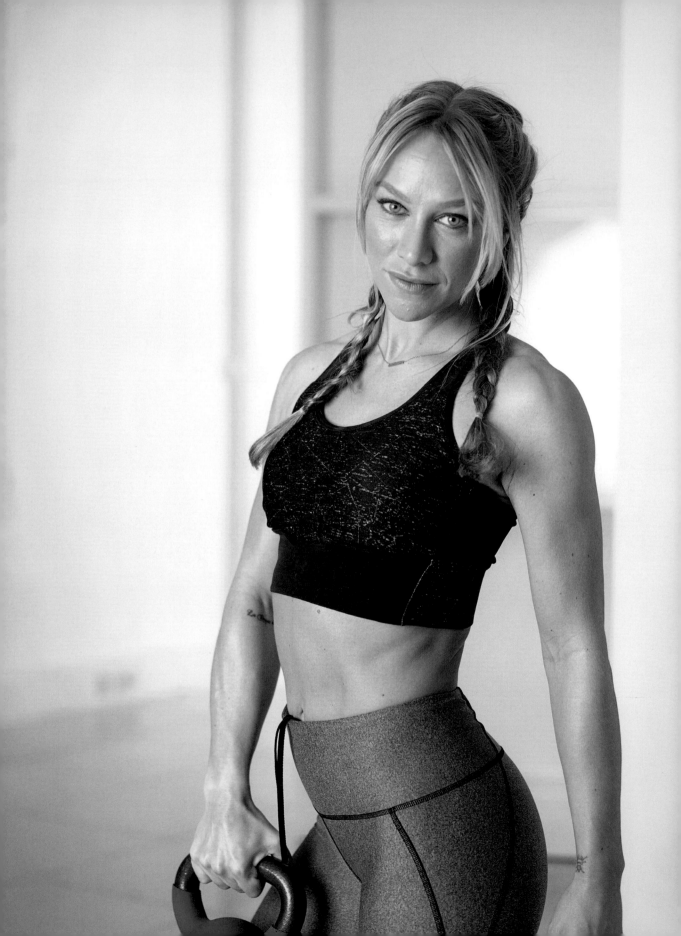

YOUR PHYSIQUE GOAL

DIET & CARDIO

CHOOSING YOUR PHYSIQUE GOAL

Please note that you do not have to choose a physique goal; you can simply use this book as a weight-lifting guide.

In Part 1 of this book, you first chose your lifting level (beginner / intermediate / advanced).

You then chose your lifting goal (endurance / hypertrophy / strength).

In this section, you can now choose the physique goal you want to accomplish...

» **Fat Loss**
» **Muscle Building (Hypertrophy)**

Strength training is strictly a performance goal.

While it might be tempting to choose multiple goals, let me be very clear right now... **You should only choose ONE goal at a time.**

Fat loss, muscle building (hypertrophy) and **strength training** require three very different approaches to both diet and training...

FAT LOSS

When it comes to a fat-loss plan, while I do encourage continued weight lifting in the endurance and / or hypertrophy ranges to help preserve muscle mass, it is very unlikely that you will actually gain muscle mass while in a fat-loss phase. This is because muscle needs fuel, aka calories, to grow, and if you are in a calorie deficit via food intake and / or cardio output, your muscle will be fighting to hang around, at best.

This is not to say that muscle gain in a fat-loss phase is impossible; it can happen, especially for beginners (this is often referred to as 'newbie gains'). However, for the majority of us, it is rare. So, while I do encourage you to keep lifting, don't be surprised if you end up looking a little less muscular and a little more slender.

My advice is to build the muscle *first*, shed the fat *later*.

MUSCLE BUILDING
(Hypertrophy)

When it comes to a muscle-building plan, you shouldn't be concerned with fat loss. In fact, if you are actively trying to gain muscle, then you will probably gain a little fat (I always do). This is because in order to fuel your training, recover from your training, and actually grow your muscle, you need to eat very well.

My advice is to build the muscle *first*, shed the fat *later*.

STRENGTH TRAINING

When it comes to a strength plan, you shouldn't be overly concerned with any physique changes. Visible muscle gain or visible fat loss may occur due to the training, but neither is your primary goal. Strength is a performance-based goal, not an aesthetic one, that's what makes it so much fun! Aim to eat healthily and be very well fuelled calorically for both your training and your recovery – don't aim to look like a health and fitness model.

Changing Goals and Long-term Training

Although I do advise you to choose a goal, stick with it and give it 100%, there may come a time when you could or even should change your goal...

For example, you shouldn't spend more than 6 months in a fat-loss phase (in my opinion). It's simply not good for your hormones or metabolic rate (not to mention your social life). At that 6-month mark, I encourage slowly easing into a muscle-building or strength-training phase for at least 6 months before re-entering fat loss.

While you can spend as long as you want in a muscle-building (hypertrophy) phase (the longer the better, in fact), there may come a time when you want to shed some fat and get a good look at what you've built underneath. And while you can spend as long as you want in a strength-building phase, there may come a time when muscle building or fat loss takes your fancy.

DIET and your Physique Goal

The specifics of your diet will depend on your fat-loss, muscle-building or strength goal (very different diets are required for each goal), but the overall nutritional rules for those who lift weights are always the same...

Your daily diet should be composed of 3 macronutrients:

1 **Proteins** (dominant macro)
2 **Fats** (the quantity will be goal dependent)
3 **Carbohydrates** (the quantity will be goal dependent)

You should also be concerned with other pivotal dietary factors:

» **Micronutrients** (vitamins and minerals from fruit and veg)
» **Fibre** (from wholegrains, fruit and veg – aka all food grown from the earth)
» **Hydration** (daily water intake)
» **Supplementation** (when and where necessary, such as omega oils for those on a lower fat diet)

CARDIO and your Physique Goal

The specifics of your cardio will depend on your fat loss, muscle building or strength goal (very different approaches to cardio are required for each goal), but cardio should be a part of any and every plan regardless of goals.

» For fat loss, it should be used as a calorie burning and / or metabolic boosting tool.
» For muscle building (hypertrophy) and strength training, it should be used as a strength, fitness and recovery tool.
» Your types, times and frequency of cardio will differ but, ultimately, cardio is a necessity for everyone.

A FAT-LOSS PHYSIQUE GOAL

If fat loss is your goal, you need to be in a calorie deficit.

A calorie deficit simply means that your body is burning (via general movement and / or exercise) more energy than it is consuming (via food). This forces your body to burn into its fat stores.

You can achieve a calorie deficit by:

» Increasing your movement (typically via cardio increase)

» Decreasing your calorie intake

» Doing a little bit of both

I recommend this third option as it ensures that you don't over-train or under-eat. Instead, you will have productive exercise sessions and a diet that you can adhere to.

The Fat-loss Diet

A typical fat-loss diet includes lean proteins (egg whites, whey protein, lean beef, chicken or fish, for example), with a constant intake of vegetables (for micronutrients and fibre), a small amount of carbohydrates (oats, rice and potato, for example) timed around training sessions (pre and / or post). The rest of the time a small amount of fats (eggs, nuts and avocado, for example) should replace carbohydrates in your meals.

While this may be a 'typical fat-loss diet', as long as you are in a calorie deficit, you can implement it however you prefer.

Go through The Food Bible (see pages 190–201) to familiarise yourself with portion sizes and check out the recipes on pages 204–234. Make sure you choose low-carb options (look out for the ⟱ symbol), unless you are on a refeed day.

Fat loss is the only goal in this book that comes with a time limit. I am happy for my clients to spend 4–24 weeks in a fat-loss phase, but after that 24-week (6-month) mark, I encourage them to slowly increase their food intake, decrease their cardio times and / or days, and allow their body to recover.

Tracking Calories and Macros

If you track calories and macros on an app (I recommend MyFitnessPal):

» **Track your daily intake for 1–2 weeks** to get an idea of your protein, fat, carbohydrate and calorie intake.

» **If you are not hitting 2g protein per 1kg of lean bodyweight** (for example, if 70kg was my leanest adult body weight, I should intake around 140g protein daily), make sure you start to work your way up to that and remember that, once there, this intake should always stay stable, regardless of your goals.

» **In terms of carbs and fats, you should be hitting 1g of both per 1kg of lean bodyweight** (so if 70kg was my leanest adult bodyweight, that would be 70g fats and 70g carbs daily).

This 2protein/1carb/1fat macro split should bring you to around about your BMR (Basal Metabolic Rate – the number of calories your body needs to function, in other words your basement calorie intake).

Once you have your 2/1/1 macro split set, look at how many calories you burn in a typical training session...

If fat loss is your goal, you should make up around 75% of these burned calories via added carbohydrates.

For example, if I burned roughly 400kcals in a typical training session, I would add 300kcals' worth of carbohydrates to my intake. I would *not* add all 400kcals of the burned calories because I want to be in a calorie deficit.

If after 2 or more weeks you plateau, you can either increase your cardio output by a small amount (5–10 minutes a session) OR decrease your fats or carbs by a small amount (5–10g).

You can do this every time you plateau for 2 or more weeks, but under no other circumstances should you increase your deficit – fat loss takes time AND you need room to manoeuvre as time passes.

Where is the basement?

I would never recommend dropping below 2g protein per 1kg lean body weight if you have ANY kind of performance OR physique goal.

In terms of fat loss, I would stop dropping fat at 0.5g per kg of bodyweight (for someone who is 70kg, this would be 35g fat) and stop dropping carbohydrates at 1g per kg of bodyweight (for someone who is 70kg, this would be 70g carbohydrates).

★ ★

If you are not someone who can be bothered to weigh out and track your food every day (hello the vast majority of the population!) then what you need is a diet plan…

★

THE FAT-LOSS DIET PLAN

Monday–Friday

Low-calorie via *low-carb* meals and snacks

BREAKFAST

CHOOSE:

1 protein option

+

1 fat option

+

1 veg option

OR

1 low-carb recipe

LUNCH

CHOOSE:

1 protein option

+

1 fat option

+

1 veg option

OR

1 low-carb recipe

DINNER

CHOOSE:

1 protein option

+

1 fat option

+

1 veg option

OR

1 low-carb recipe

SNACK 1

CHOOSE:

1 protein option

+IF YOU LIKE+

1 veg option

SNACK 2

CHOOSE:

1 protein option

+IF YOU LIKE+

1 veg option

POST WEIGHTLIFTING

If you have just finished a weight-lifting session, replace your next low-carb meal with:

1 protein option

+

1 carb option

+

1 veg option

OR

1 high-carb recipe

MEN

Men need to follow the above structure but:

» Replace the 2 daily snacks with 2 daily low-carb meals

» Implement a 3rd snack (low-carb meal)

This will ensure men hit the appropriate calorie count.

The post-training, high-carb meal swap applies to men as well.

THE FAT-LOSS DIET PLAN

Saturday + Sunday

Two refeed days via carbohydrate increase to aid the inevitable hormonal, metabolic and glycogenic adaptations of a fat-loss diet

BREAKFAST
CHOOSE:
1 protein option
+
1 carb option
+
1 veg option
OR
1 high-carb recipe

....

SNACK 1
CHOOSE:
1 protein option
+IF YOU LIKE+
1 veg option

LUNCH
CHOOSE:
1 protein option
+
1 carb option
+
1 veg option
OR
1 high-carb recipe

....

SNACK 2
CHOOSE:
1 protein option
+IF YOU LIKE+
1 veg option

DINNER
CHOOSE:
1 protein option
+
1 carb option
+
1 veg option
OR
1 high-carb recipe

....

SNACK 3
CHOOSE:
1 carb option
+IF YOU LIKE+
1 veg option

MEN
Men need to follow the above structure but:

» Replace 2 of the daily snacks with 2 daily high-carb meals

» Implement a 4th snack (high-carb ⏫ meal)

This will ensure men hit the appropriate refeed calorie count

The post-training, high-carb meal swap applies to men as well.

Please note: I am happy for you to spend up to 24 weeks (6 months) total in a fat-loss phase, but after that time, you should slowly increase your food intake, decrease your cardio, and allow your body to recover.

FAT-LOSS CARDIO

If fat loss is your goal, I would like you to:

» Continue lifting 4–6 days a week

In one of the following 2 ranges:

» Endurance

AND / OR

» Hypertrophy

When to do your cardio?

» Fasted in the morning (hours pre lift)

OR

» Post lift (immediately post lift or hours post lift)

How often?

» 4–6 days a week

Fat-loss cardio should be a good mix of:

» High Intensity Interval Training (HIIT)

» Low or Moderate Intensity Steady State (LISS or MISS)

The reason I want you to perform your cardio either fasted first thing in the morning **OR** post-lift is to make sure that you are doing your lifting at a time when you have optimum energy.

Lifting is harder than cardio and requires more mental and physical energy. If you get your cardio done and out of the way first thing in the morning, you can then fuel up throughout the day and give 100% to your lifting later on.

If you aren't able to do your cardio first thing in the morning, then make sure you do it after lifting.

The lifting session should always be your primary concern when it comes to training – lifting requires no less than 100% mental and physical attention. Cardio, on the other hand, is simply another tool to burn calories and / or stay fit.

How long can I do the Fat-loss Cardio Plan?

You'll notice that your weekly cardio plan is only 4 weeks.

This is because I usually recommend implementing a fat-loss phase for between 4 weeks (minimum) and 24 weeks (maximum).

If you choose to continue with your fat-loss plan for more than 4 weeks, I suggest you continue with the week 4 instructions for as long as possible.

However, if you find that you plateau for more than 2 weeks, you may add:

» 2 minutes of HIIT

AND

» 5 minutes of LISS / MISS

BUT there is absolutely a cap when it comes to cardio.

I personally recommend capping:

» HIIT at 45 minutes total

» LISS and MISS at 1 hour total

» 6 cardio sessions weekly MAX

Fat loss is the only goal in this book that comes with a time limit. I am happy for you to spend 4–24 weeks in a fat-loss phase, but after that 24-week (6-month) mark, I encourage you to slowly increase your food intake, decrease your cardio and allow your body to recover.

After a few months of consuming more calories and performing less cardio (ideally in a muscle-building or strength phase) I am happy for you to go back into a fat-loss phase.

This cyclical approach to fat loss is highly successful, perfectly healthy and surprisingly enjoyable.

If fat loss is your goal, understand that it is NOT easy and requires no less than 100% commitment to BOTH your diet and cardio plans.

THE FAT-LOSS CARDIO PLAN

WEEK

MONDAY Lower Body
HIIT CARDIO – 20 minutes
Burpees
or
Any cardio machine (resistance added)
x 30 seconds **100% effort**
Rest: 90 seconds
Repeat: x 10 times
Total: 20 minutes

....

TUESDAY Upper Body
LISS CARDIO – 20 minutes
Outdoor power walk (include some uphill if possible)
or
Swim
or
Any cardio machine (slight resistance)
Total: 20 minutes

....

WEDNESDAY Back/Core
MISS CARDIO – 20 minutes
Uphill / Incline / Steep power walk
or
Hard swim
or
Any cardio machine (resistance added)
Total: 20 minutes

THURSDAY Lower Body
HIIT CARDIO – 20 minutes
Burpees
or
Any cardio machine (resistance added)
x 30 seconds **100% effort**
Rest: 90 seconds
Repeat: x 10 times
Total: 20 minutes

....

FRIDAY Upper Body
LISS CARDIO – 20 minutes
Outdoor power walk (include some uphill if possible)
or
Swim
or
Any cardio machine (slight resistance)
Total: 20 minutes

....

SATURDAY Back/Core
MISS CARDIO – 20 minutes
Uphill / Incline / Steep power walk
or
Hard swim
or
Any cardio machine (resistance added)
Total: 20 minutes

SUNDAY Rest Day

THE FAT-LOSS CARDIO PLAN

WEEK

MONDAY Lower Body

HIIT CARDIO – 22 minutes

Mountain Climbers
or
Any cardio machine (resistance added)
x 30 seconds **100% effort**
Rest: 90 seconds
Repeat: x 11 times
Total: 22 minutes

....

TUESDAY Upper Body

LISS CARDIO – 25 minutes

Outdoor power walk (include some uphill if possible)
or
Swim
or
Any cardio machine (slight resistance)
Total: 25 minutes

....

WEDNESDAY Back/Core

MISS CARDIO – 25 minutes

Uphill / Incline / Steep power walk
or
Hard swim
or
Any cardio machine (resistance added)
Total: 25 minutes

THURSDAY Lower Body

HIIT CARDIO – 22 minutes

Mountain Climbers
or
Any cardio machine (resistance added)
x 30 seconds **100% effort**
Rest: 90 seconds
Repeat: x 11 times
Total: 22 minutes

....

FRIDAY Upper Body

LISS CARDIO – 25 minutes

Outdoor power walk (include some uphill if possible)
or
Swim
or
Any cardio machine (slight resistance)
Total: 25 minutes

....

SATURDAY Back/Core

MISS CARDIO – 25 minutes

Uphill / Incline / Steep power walk
or
Hard swim
or
Any cardio machine (resistance added)
Total: 25 minutes

SUNDAY Rest Day

THE FAT-LOSS CARDIO PLAN

WEEK

3

MONDAY Lower Body
HIIT CARDIO – 24 minutes
Squat Jumps
or
Any cardio machine (resistance added)
x 30 seconds **100% effort**
Rest: 90 seconds
Repeat: x 12 times
Total: 24 minutes

....

TUESDAY Upper Body
LISS CARDIO – 30 minutes
Outdoor power walk (include some uphill if possible)
or
Swim
or
Any cardio machine (slight resistance)
Total: 30 minutes

....

WEDNESDAY Back/Core
MISS CARDIO – 30 minutes
Uphill / Incline / Steep power walk
or
Hard swim
or
Any cardio machine (resistance added)
Total: 30 minutes

THURSDAY Lower Body
HIIT CARDIO – 24 minutes
Squat Jumps
or
Any cardio machine (resistance added)
x 30 seconds **100% effort**
Rest: 90 seconds
Repeat: x 12 times
Total: 24 minutes

....

FRIDAY Upper Body
LISS CARDIO – 30 minutes
Outdoor power walk (include some uphill if possible)
or
Swim
or
Any cardio machine (slight resistance)
Total: 30 minutes

....

SATURDAY Back/Core
MISS CARDIO – 30 minutes
Uphill / Incline / Steep power walk
or
Hard swim
or
Any cardio machine (resistance added)
Total: 30 minutes

SUNDAY Rest Day

THE FAT-LOSS CARDIO PLAN

WEEK

4

MONDAY Lower Body
HIIT CARDIO – 26 minutes

Burpees
or
Any cardio machine (resistance added)
x 30 seconds **100% effort**
Rest: 90 seconds
Repeat: x 13 times
Total: 26 minutes

....

TUESDAY Upper Body
LISS CARDIO – 35 minutes

Outdoor walk (include some uphill if possible)
or
Swim
or
Any cardio machine (slight resistance)
Total: 35 minutes

....

WEDNESDAY Back/Core
MISS CARDIO – 35 minutes

Uphill / Incline / Steep power walk
or
Hard swim
or
Any cardio machine (resistance added)
Total: 35 minutes

THURSDAY Lower Body
HIIT CARDIO – 26 minutes

Burpees
or
Any cardio machine (resistance added)
x 30 seconds **100% effort**
Rest: 90 seconds
Repeat: x 13 times
Total: 26 minutes

....

FRIDAY Upper Body
LISS CARDIO – 35 minutes

Outdoor walk (include some uphill if possible)
or
Swim
or
Any cardio machine (slight resistance)
Total: 35 minutes

....

SATURDAY Back/Core
MISS CARDIO – 35 minutes

Uphill / Incline / Steep power walk
or
Hard swim
or
Any cardio machine (resistance added)
Total: 35 minutes

SUNDAY Rest Day

A MUSCLE-BUILDING (HYPERTROPHY) PHYSIQUE GOAL

If muscle building (hypertrophy) is your goal, as well as the muscle-building diet and cardio plans that are detailed below, you will need to follow a hypertrophy weight-lifting plan (see pages 30–165).

The Muscle-building (Hypertrophy) Diet

With a muscle building (hypertrophy) goal, you need to be in a calorie surplus so that your body can add to itself. Think about it, how are you going to push your body to grow if you don't feed it to do so?

As well as calories, you also need to be aware of how to structure your specific macronutrients, in order to optimise your:

>> Training

>> Recovery

>> Gains

Essentially, protein and carbohydrates are going to be your new best friends.

Meals should be high in protein (for example, egg whites, whey protein, meat, chicken and fish) with omnipresent vegetables and carbohydrates (for example, oats, cereals, bread, rice, pasta or potato) every day, especially around training (pre and post). A small amount of fats (for example, eggs, nuts, oils or avocado) should accompany carbohydrates in your daily meals.

Go through The Food Bible (see pages 190–201) to familiarise yourself with portion sizes and check out the recipes on pages 204–234.

Make sure you choose some Gains options (look out for the ⌾ symbol).

Bearing in mind that you need to be in a calorie surplus, you might want to look into using a protein powder that is a mass gainer.

If you want to build muscle, it is pivotal that you eat a big meal before training AND after training, for energy, recovery and results.

Tracking Calories and Macros

If you track calories and macros on an app (I recommend MyFitnessPal):

>> **Track your daily intake for 1–2 weeks** to get an idea of your protein, fat, carbohydrate and calorie intake.

>> **If you are not hitting 2g protein per 1kg of lean bodyweight** (for example, if 70kg was my leanest adult body weight, I should intake around 140g protein daily), make sure you start to work your way up to that and remember that, once there, this intake should always stay stable, regardless of your goals.

>> **In terms of carbs and fats, you should be hitting 1g of both per 1kg of lean bodyweight** (so if 70kg was my leanest adult bodyweight, that would be 70g carbs and 70g fats daily).

This 2protein/1carb/1fat macro split should bring you to around about your BMR (Basal Metabolic Rate – the number of calories your body needs to function, in other words your basement calorie intake).

Once you have your 2/1/1 macro split set, look at how many calories you burn in a typical training session...

If muscle building (hypertrophy) is your goal, you need to make up 150% of these burned calories via added carbohydrates. For example, if I burned roughly 400kcals in a typical training session, I would add 600kcals' worth of **carbohydrates** to my intake (there are 4kcals in 1g of carb, so 600kcals is 150g carbs).

If after 2 or more weeks you plateau, you can increase your carbs by 30g (120kcals) and see if your weight increases.

You can do this every time you plateau for 2 or more weeks.

» I would start to work your way up to 4–5g carbohydrates per 1kg of lean bodyweight. For example, if I weighed 70kg I should work my way up to an intake of 280–350g carbohydrates daily.

» Don't panic if you start to gain some body fat, this is very normal when in a muscle-building phase and calorie surplus.

However, if you gain too much body fat too quickly, simply stop increasing your carbohydrates for the time being and see if your body stabilises. If it doesn't and you want to drop a little body fat, deduct 5–10g from your daily carbohydrate or fat intake and then see how your body responds. You can repeat this process if need be, but I encourage you to accept that increased muscle does invite increased body fat.

Where is the ceiling?

If you are actively trying to gain and grow, it's unlikely you'll reach a point at which you have to cap your intake – gaining muscle is a hard thing to do!

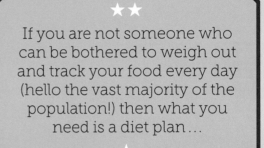

★ ★

If you are not someone who can be bothered to weigh out and track your food every day (hello the vast majority of the population!) then what you need is a diet plan...

★

THE MUSCLE-BUILDING DIET PLAN

Monday–Sunday

Protein, carbohydrate and fat balanced meals for training fuel, recovery and muscle growth

BREAKFAST
CHOOSE:
1 protein option
+
1 carb
+
1 fat option
+
1 veg option
OR
1 Gains recipe

LUNCH
CHOOSE:
1 protein option
+
1 carb
+
1 fat option
+
1 veg option
OR
1 Gains recipe

DINNER
CHOOSE:
1 protein option
+
1 carb
+
1 fat option
+
1 veg option
OR
1 Gains recipe

....

SNACK 1
CHOOSE:
1 protein option
+IF YOU LIKE+
1 veg option

SNACK 2
CHOOSE:
1 protein option
+IF YOU LIKE+
1 veg option

MEN

Men need to follow the above structure but:

» Replace the 2 daily snacks with 2 daily Gains meals instead

» Implement a 3rd snack (◉ Gains meal)

This will ensure men hit the appropriate calorie count.

If you find that you plateau at a certain weight or physique but your training is on point, you may well need to add to your daily food intake … I would advise adding:

» 1 Gains recipe to your daily intake, ideally before or after your training

MUSCLE-BUILDING (HYPERTROPHY) CARDIO

If muscle building (hypertrophy) is your goal, I would like you to:

» Lift 4–6 days a week in the hypertrophy range

Only implementing **10-minute HIIT sessions**:

» Immediately post lift

» Every other training day (2–3 times a week), ideally on lower body days

You don't want to overdo cardio if muscle building is your goal, as you need to focus on maintaining high energy for your lifts and on your recovery afterwards. You also want your caloric intake to be going towards muscle building, both in the gym and after, and not towards cardio energy output.

The reason I want you to perform your cardio immediately post lift is to make sure you have optimum energy for your lift, which is harder and requires more mental and physical energy than cardio does.

If you get your lift done first and give it 100%, you can roll on to cardio without having to worry about lifting heavy weights afterwards.

A lot of people would not recommend doing any cardio when you're in a muscle-building phase, but I disagree. Cardiovascular exercise is healthy and, when done in the right amounts and ranges, can assist pretty much any training or physique goal. Short, sharp, intermittent HIIT days work nicely with a muscle-building goal and a hypertrophy lifting plan.

How long can I do the Muscle-building (Hypertrophy) Plan?

There is no time limit to a muscle-building plan. However, if you find you plateau at a certain weight or physique, you will need to do one (or several) of the following:

» Increase your calories (ideally via increased carbohydrates)

» Play around with your nutrient timing (pre- and post-training protein, carbohydrate and calorie increases)

» Increase your training sets, reps and / or weight ranges (increased volume and / or intensity)

» Potentially switch your hypertrophy to strength training for a period of time, before switching back to hypertrophy

---

MONDAY + THURSDAY
Lower Body
HIIT CARDIO – 10 minutes
Burpees
or
Any cardio machine (resistance added)
x 30 seconds **100% effort**
Rest: 90 seconds
Repeat: x 5 times
Total: 10 minutes

A STRENGTH-TRAINING GOAL

If strength is your goal, as well as the strength diet and cardio plans that are detailed below, you will need to follow a strength weight-lifting plan for 4–6 days a week (see pages 30–165).

The Strength-training Diet

With a strength goal, you need to make sure you are eating either at maintenance calories or in a calorie surplus so that your body can perform and recover sufficiently.

You also need to be aware of how to structure your specific macronutrients, in order to optimise your:

» Training
» Recovery
» Gains

Essentially, protein and carbohydrates are going to be your new best friends.

Meals should be high in protein (for example, egg whites, whey protein, meat, chicken and fish) with omnipresent vegetables and carbohydrates (for example, oats, cereal, bread, rice, pasta or potato) every day, especially around training (pre and post). A small amount of fats (for example, eggs, nuts, oils and avocado) should accompany carbohydrates in your daily meals.

Go through The Food Bible (see pages 190–201) to familiarise yourself with portion sizes and check out the recipes on pages 204–234. Make sure you choose some Gains options (look out for the ⊙ symbol).

Make sure you always eat a big meal *before* training AND *after* training, as it is pivotal to your session, recovery and increased strength results.

Tracking Calories and Macros

If you track calories and macros on an app (I recommend MyFitnessPal):

» **Track your daily intake for 1–2 weeks** to get an idea of your protein, fat, carbohydrate and calorie intake

» **If you are not hitting 2g protein per 1kg of lean bodyweight** (for example, if 70kg was my leanest adult body weight, I should intake around 140g protein daily), make sure you start to work your way up to that and remember that, once there, this intake should always stay stable, regardless of your goals.

» **In terms of carbs and fats, you should be hitting 1g of both per 1kg of lean bodyweight** (so if 70kg was my leanest adult bodyweight, that would be 70g carbs and 70g fats daily).

This 2protein/1carb/1fat macro split should bring you to around about your BMR (Basal Metabolic Rate – the number of calories your body needs to function, in other words your basement calorie intake).

Once you have your 2/1/1 macro split set, look at how many calories you burn in a typical training session…

If strength is your goal, you need to make up 100% of these burned calories via added carbohydrates. For example, if I burned roughly 400kcals in a typical training session, I would add 400kcals' worth of carbohydrates to my intake (there are 4kcals in 1g of carb, so 400kcals is 100g carbs).

If you instinctively feel that you can and / or should increase your food intake in order to increase your strength-training abilities, you can increase your carbs by 30g (120kcals) and see if your training benefits. You can do this every time you feel you need to.

» I would start to work your way up to 4–5g carbohydrates per 1kg of lean bodyweight (for example, if I weighed 70kg I should work my way up to an intake of 280–350g carbohydrates daily).

» Don't panic if you start to gain some body fat, this is very normal when in a calorie surplus.

However, if you gain too much body fat too quickly, simply stop increasing your carbohydrates for the time being and see if your body stabilises. If it doesn't and you want to drop a little body fat, deduct 5–10g from your daily carbohydrate or fat intake and then see how your body responds.

Where is the ceiling?

If you are actively trying to increase strength and perform better, you might not reach a point at which you cap your intake – increasing strength is a hard thing to do!

★★
If you are not someone who can be bothered to weigh out and track your food every day (hello the vast majority of the population!) then what you need is a diet plan…
★

THE STRENGTH DIET PLAN

Monday–Sunday

Protein, carbohydrate and fat balanced meals for performance and recovery

BREAKFAST

CHOOSE:

1 protein option

+

1 carb

+

1 fat option

+

1 veg option

OR

1 Gains recipe

....

SNACK 1

CHOOSE:

1 protein option

+IF YOU LIKE+

1 veg option

LUNCH

CHOOSE:

1 protein option

+

1 carb

+

1 fat option

+

1 veg option

OR

1 Gains recipe

....

SNACK 2

CHOOSE:

1 protein option

+IF YOU LIKE+

1 veg option

DINNER

CHOOSE:

1 protein option

+

1 carb

+

1 fat option

+

1 veg option

OR

1 Gains recipe

....

MEN

Men need to follow the above structure but:

» Replace the 2 daily snacks with 2 daily Gains meals instead

» Implement a 3rd snack (Gains meal)

This will ensure men hit the appropriate calorie count

STRENGTH CARDIO

If strength is your goal, I would like you to:

» Lift 4–6 days a week in the strength range (remember that less is more with strength training – recovery is key!)

Only implementing 20–30 minutes:

» Low-impact cardio (swimming, rowing, cross trainer etc) **AND**

» Low Intensity Steady State (LISS) cardio

When to do your cardio?

» 2–3 days a week

» On your rest days **OR**

» Immediately post lift (ideally on lower body days)

Recovery is key for strength and while a little LISS can aid recovery, too much of it can hinder recovery.

The reason I want you to perform your cardio on your rest days OR immediately post lift is to make sure you have optimum energy for your lift, which is harder and requires more mental and physical energy. If you get your lift done first and give it 100%, you can then roll on to cardio without having to worry about squatting a baby elephant afterwards.

A lot of people don't recommend any cardio when in a strength phase, but I disagree. Cardiovascular exercise it healthy and, when done in the right amounts and ranges, can assist pretty much any training goal.

Low-impact, low-intensity cardio can work nicely alongside a strength training plan.

How long can I do the Strength-building Cardio Plan?

There is no time limit to a strength-building plan. However, if you find you hit your limit on a certain lift and you cannot get past it, you will need to do one (or several) of the following:

» Increase your calories (ideally via increased carbohydrates)

» Play around with your nutrient timing (pre- and post-training protein, carbohydrate and calorie increases)

» Implement a deload week (deliberately decrease your training output – frequency, volume and / or intensity)

» Add in some hypertrophy accessory work (additional lifts that will assist your strength performance, such as a leg press to help improve a squat)

MONDAY + THURSDAY
Lower Body
LISS CARDIO – 20–30 minutes MAX
Swim
or
Any LOW-IMPACT cardio machine (slight resistance)
Total: 20–30 minutes MAX

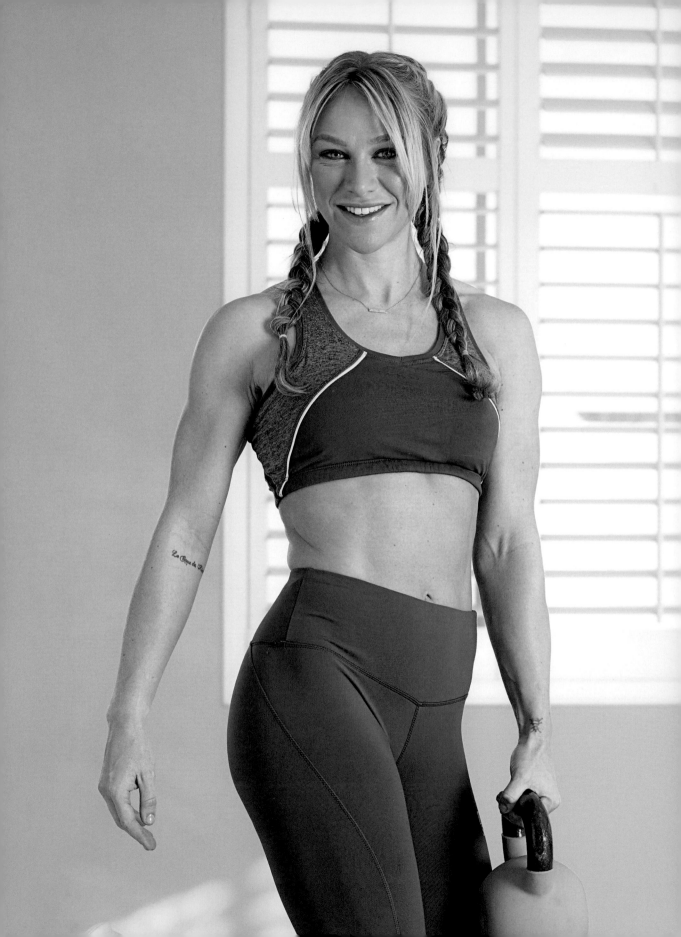

THE
FOOD BIBLE
& RECIPES

THE FOOD BIBLE

PROTEIN

Every option listed is 1 'standard' portion of protein.

All proteins marked in **red** are higher calories owing to a higher fat content. If you choose one of these as your protein portion, it will also count as your fat portion.

Anything in **green** is a personal brand suggestion. These suggestions are not endorsed – they are simply based on my years of tracking calories and macros and finding the most 'bang for my buck' foods.

DAIRY

PROTEIN	EASE	GRAMS
Eat Lean Protein Cheese	80g	80g
Greek Yoghurt Plain 0% or Plain full-fat	200g pot or 200g pot	200g or 200g
Cottage Cheese Plain fat-free or Plain full-fat	200g tub or 200g tub	200g or 200g

FISH

PROTEIN	EASE	GRAMS
Cod	1 small fillet	Approx. 120g
Crayfish	1 small packet	Typically 150g
Haddock	1 small fillet	Approx. 120g
King Scallops	2 large	Approx. 120g
Lobster	1 small	1 small
Mussels	1 small bowl	Approx. 150g
Prawns	1 small packet	Approx. 150g
Salmon Fillet or Smoked or Tinned	1 small fillet or 4 small slices or 1 small tin	Approx. 120g or Approx. 80g or Typically 105g
Scallops	1 small packet/bowl	Approx. 150g
Sole	1 small fillet	Approx. 120g
Squid	1 small packet/bowl	Approx. 150g
Tuna Steak or Tinned in water or brine or Tinned in sunflower or olive oil	1 small steak or 1 tin or 1 tin	Approx. 120g or Typically 110g (drained) or Typically 110g (drained)

MEAT

PROTEIN	EASE	GRAMS
Beef 5% mince or 10% mince or 15% mince or Fillet steak	200g packet or 175g packet or 150g packet or 1 small	200g or 175g or 150g or Approx. 200g
Chicken Breast (skinless/boneless) or Chipolatas (Heck Chicken Chipolatas)	1 breast or 3 chipolatas	Approx. 125g
Duck (skinless/boneless)	1 small breast	Approx. 125g
Pork Bacon Sausage	2 slices 1 sausage 2 sausages	
Turkey Bacon or Breast (skinless/boneless) or Breast Mince	3 slices or 1 small breast or 100g packet	Approx. 125g or 100g

OTHER

PROTEIN	EASE	GRAMS
Eggs	2 small or 4 small	
Egg Whites	8 large or 300g	Approx. 300g
Quorn (mince/pieces) Quorn	100g	100g
Soy (Tofu etc)	100g packet	100g
Soy Yoghurt (Plain)	300g pot	300g
Whey Protein Powder	1 serving	Typically 25–30g

Remember that protein is the
macro that will mend the
muscle tissue you have torn in
training. It is vital to recovery
and physique results.

FAT

Every option listed is 1 'standard' portion of fat. Don't forget that your specific fat requirements will depend on your specific aesthetic goal (see pages 170–9, 180–3 and 184–7).

All fats marked in **red** are higher calorie owing to a higher protein content. If you choose one of these as your fat portion, it will also count as your protein portion.

Anything in **green** is a personal brand suggestion. These suggestions are not endorsed – they are simply based on my years of tracking calories and macros and finding the most 'bang for my buck' foods.

While protein and carbs have 4kcals per 1g, fats have more than double that – 9kcals per 1g. For this reason, you want to make sure you consume fats in moderation, while remembering that they are a macronutrient and are pivotal to the health and function of the human body.

DAIRY

FAT	EASE	GRAMS
Brie	2 knife smears	Approx. 40g
Butter	1 level tbsp	Approx. 15g
Camembert	2 knife smears	Approx. 40g
Cheddar	1 small handful of grated	Approx. 30g
Cottage Cheese Full-fat	100g tub or 200g tub	100g or 200g
Cream Double Single Soured	2 level tbsp 4 level tbsp 4 level tbsp	Approx. 30ml Approx. 60ml Approx. 60ml
Cream Cheese Full-fat	2 level tbsp	Approx. 30g
Edam	1 small handful of grated	Approx. 30g
Emmental	1 small handful of grated	Approx. 30g
Feta	1 small handful of crumbled	Approx. 30g
Halloumi	1 slice	Typically 30g
Mozzarella	1 small handful of torn or grated	Approx. 30g
Parmesan	2 level tbsp of grated	Approx. 30g
Yoghurt Plain Greek full-fat Fage	100g pot or 200g pot	100g or 200g

FISH

FAT	EASE	GRAMS
Mackerel	1 fillet	Typically 100g
Salmon Fillet or Smoked or Tinned	1 small fillet or 4 small slices or 1 small tin	Approx. 120g or Approx. 80g or Typically 105g
Sardines	2 small	Typically 110g
Tinned Tuna in sunflower or olive oil	1 tin	Typically 110g (drained)

MEAT

FAT	EASE	GRAMS
Beef 5% mince or 10% mince or 15% mince or Fillet steak	200g packet or 175g packet or 150g packet or 1 small	200g or 175g or 150g or Approx. 200g
Pork Bacon Sausage	2 slices 1 sausage 2 sausages	Approx. 30g

OTHER

FAT	EASE	GRAMS
Avocado	½ small	Approx. 60g
Cacao Nibs	1 level tbsp	Approx. 15g
Chocolate (90% cocoa solids)	2 squares	Approx. 25g
Eggs	2 small or 4 small	
Mayonnaise	1 level tbsp	Approx.15g
Nuts (all)	1 small palm size	Approx. 20g
Nut butters Peanut Meridian Almond Meridian Cashew Meridian	1 level tbsp	Approx. 15g
Hummus	2 level tbsp	Approx. 30g
Oil (all)	1 level tbsp	Approx. 15g
Olives (all)	1 handful	Approx. 75g
Pesto (all)	1 level tbsp	Approx. 15g
Seeds (all)	1 small palm size	Approx. 20g
Tahini Meridian	1 level tbsp	Approx. 15g

CARBOHYDRATES

Every option listed is 1 'standard' portion of carbohydrate. Don't forget that your specific carbohydrate requirements will depend on your specific aesthetic goal (see pages 170–9, 180–3 and 184–7).

Anything in **green** is a personal brand suggestion. These suggestions are not endorsed – they are simply based on my years of tracking calories and macros and finding the most 'bang for my buck' foods.

FRUITS/STARCHY VEG

CARBOHYDRATE	EASE	GRAMS
Fruit (any)	1 small portion	Approx. 50g
Legumes and all pulses (beans/peas/lentils etc.)	¼ tin	Approx. 100g
Potatoes and all starchy veg (parsnips/plantain/pumpkin/peas/corn etc.)	1 small serving	Approx. 150g

GRAINS/PASTA

CARBOHYDRATE	EASE	GRAMS
Couscous	1 small bowl	Approx. 40g (dry) or Approx. 100g (cooked)
Granola (any Plain)	1 handful (dry)	Approx. 30g (dry)
Muesli (any Plain)	1 small bowl (dry)	Approx. 30g (dry)
Oats (any Plain)	3 level tbsp or 1 small bowl (dry)	Approx. 30g (dry)
Pasta (Wholegrain)	1 small bowl	Approx. 40g (dry) or Approx. 80g (cooked)
Popcorn (Plain)	1 small bag or 2 large handfuls or 25g kernels	Approx. 25g
Puffed Rice Cereal (any Plain)	1 small bowl (dry)	Approx. 30g (dry)
Quinoa	1 small bowl	Approx. 40g (dry) or Approx. 100g (cooked)
Rice (Wholegrain)	1 small bowl	Approx. 40g (dry) or Approx. 80g (cooked)
Rice Cakes	3 rice cakes	Approx. 10g each
Taco Shells	2 shells	Approx. 15g each
Weetabix (Plain)	2 biscuits	Approx. 40g

BREADS

CARBOHYDRATE	EASE	GRAMS
Bagel (Plain wholegrain)	½ normal or 1 thin	Approx. 45g or Approx. 45g
Bread (any wholegrain)	1 slice	Approx. 40–50g
Crumpet (any)	1 normal or 2 thin	Approx. 55g or Approx. 50g
English Muffin	1 small	Approx. 60g
Pitta Bread (any wholegrain)	1 standard size	Approx. 50g
Scotch/American Pancake (any plain)	1 small	Approx. 40g
Tortilla Wrap (Plain small wholegrain)	1 small	Approx. 40g

OTHER

CARBOHYDRATE	EASE	GRAMS
Honey	2 tbsp	Approx. 30g

VEGETABLES

Try to include non-starchy vegetables in all of your meals as they are essential to both your internal and external health.

Vegetables contain **micronutrients**, aka vitamins and minerals, that our bodies need to survive and maintain optimum health – not to mention other pivotal substances such as **fibre**.

Veg are very low calorie and, due to their high fibre content, will keep you feeling fuller for longer. This particular point is one to keep in mind if you are in a fat-loss phase specifically.

I have listed the most common non-starchy veg. However, if there are any missing from the below list, the same rules apply:

1 'standard' portion = 1 large handful

» All green leaves (lettuce/spinach/rocket etc.)
» Asparagus
» Aubergine
» Bean Sprouts
» Beetroot
» Broccoli
» Cabbage (savoy/white/red/kale/ brussels sprouts/pak choi etc.)
» Cauliflower
» Celery
» Courgette
» Cucumber (fresh/pickled etc.)
» Green Beans
» Leeks
» Mushrooms (any)
» Okra
» Onions (white/red/pickled etc)
» Peppers (any)
» Radishes
» Tomatoes (cherry/vine/plum/ chopped/tinned/passata etc.)

ADDITIONS TO MEALS AND SNACKS

Your meals and / or snacks never have to be bland.

Feel free to use any of the ingredients listed below in or alongside your meals and / or snacks.

All **green** notes are my personal brand suggestions.
These suggestions are not endorsed – they are simply based on my years of tracking calories and macros
and finding the most 'bang for my buck' foods.

Additions to meals

» Fry Light cooking spray (any)
» salt/pepper/herbs/spices
» chilli peppers (any)
» 1 tsp lemon / lime juice
» 1 clove garlic / 1 tsp chopped garlic
» 1 tsp soy sauce (any)
» 1 tsp reduced sugar ketchup
» 1 tsp vinegar (any)
» 1 tsp mustard (any)
» 1 stock cube (any)
» 1 tsp gravy granules (any)
» 1 tsp hot sauce Tabasco
» 1 tsp Sweet Freedom Choc Shot (any)
» 1 tsp sugar-free syrup (any)

DRINKS

I want women who follow this book to be aiming to drink
4 litres of water daily. Men should be aiming for 5 litres daily.

However, please feel free to work your way up to this amount
over a period of weeks if you need to.

I recommend allowing yourself a couple of hot drinks
in the morning, while sipping on a 1-litre bottle of water
into the early afternoon. Repeat this process mid-afternoon
into early evening and, hey presto, you have achieved
your water intake for the day.

Drinks marked in **red** count towards your daily water intake.

DRINK	PORTION
Diet Drinks	1 daily
Caffeinated Hot Drinks (Tea / Coffee etc.)	Up to 2 daily (morning/afternoon)
Decaffeinated Hot Drinks (Decaffeinated Coffee / Herbal Tea etc.)	Unlimited
Dairy Milk (any) OR Non-dairy Milks (any)	1 tbsp to be used in your 2 daily caffeinated hot drinks

SUPPLEMENTS

I recommend that you try to get 100% of your nutritional needs from the food that you eat. However, there are benefits to taking a few specific supplements.

Here is my list of recommendations:

›› Protein Supplements

I have a sweet tooth and protein is my dominant macro, no matter what phase I am in (fat loss or muscle building). Because of this, I usually have 1 protein supplement a day, be it a bar or a powder – usually a bar immediately post-workout to get some protein in my body ASAP, or I make protein mug cake late at night (protein + water + 2 minutes in the microwave) to ease my sweet tooth.

If you have a fat loss goal, try to go for the lower calorie, lower carb, lower fat protein sups that have a good hit of whey (a great complete protein source).

If you have a muscle building or strength goal, you have a bit more choice and freedom when selecting your protein supplements. Mass gainers can be really useful when it comes to hitting high calorie, high protein and high carb requirements, especially around training (pre and post), and there are some great supplemental foods on the market too.

›› Multivitamins

Micronutrients are the vitamins and minerals that our bodies need in order to survive and maintain optimum physical health. You should be getting these micros from your daily food intake, but most people are deficient in a few. Taking a good-quality, clinically trialled multivit can have a hugely positive impact on both your internal and external health.

›› Omega Oils

I take omega oils daily after all my meals. They reduce inflammation (which is perfect for those who train hard) and support organ health. I saw my digestion improve when I began taking them. In my opinion, these sups are a daily must.

›› Probiotics

Although it was recently proven that dairy has little-to-no impact on your gut health, clinically trialled probiotic pills have been proven to have a huge impact on your gut health and immune system. Start small – don't go for something extra strength and don't exceed the recommended dosage, as your GI tract can take a little while to adjust to probiotics.

» BCAAs (Branch Chain Amino Acids)

BCAAs (branch chain amino acids – aka complete proteins) are appropriate for those with fat loss, muscle building and / or strength goals. Pre-, intra- and/or post-workout, this supplement can help protect your muscle when you're working at 100%. It will also optimise recovery.

They're also a great option for those of you who like sugary drinks, as they come in flavoured powder form to mix with water.

» Creatine

This supplement is ideal for those wanting to build muscle and is good for strength training fans as well. Creatine can give your muscles that added oomph when it comes to training, improving high-intensity performance and encouraging muscle growth.

This is NOT a steroid and it will NOT make you 'bulky'. It is a substance that occurs naturally in our bodies and taking a daily supplement of creatine can greatly improve your strength training.

» Caffeine

A strong cup of coffee will do just as well, but if you want a pre-workout energy boost, 'pre-workouts' can help with this.

However, try to find one that has been tested by Informed-Sport (a global quality assurance programme for sports nutrition products), this way, you're reducing the risk of a crazy buzz (it may sound fun but, believe me, it does not give you a better training session!).

» CBD

Cannabidiol is a natural, non-psychoactive, safe and very much legal compound that comes from the hemp plant.

CBD impacts the human body's endocannabinoid system, affecting the central nervous and immune systems, easing inflammation, pain, oxidative stress, physical stress, mental stress and even nausea.

CBD comes in oil, powder and pill form and is usually (although not always) recommended as a single dose in the morning and evening. This product is very new to the supplement market but, so far, it is very highly rated among both the health and fitness and longevity communities.

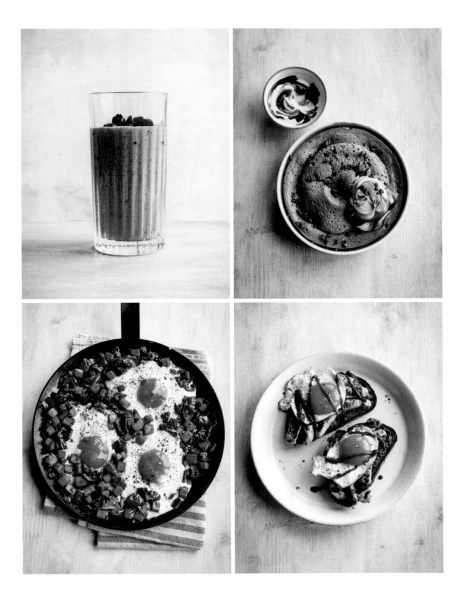

BREAKFASTS

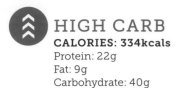

HIGH CARB

CALORIES: 334kcals
Protein: 22g
Fat: 9g
Carbohydrate: 40g

Berry Blast

This shake will get you off to a VERY healthy start indeed!

HIGH CARB

1 large handful / 1 cup frozen berries (or 1 handful fresh strawberries and 1 handful fresh blueberries)
1 large handful / 1 sachet oats (typically 30g)
170g 0% Greek yoghurt (typically 1 small pot) (Fage Total)
approx. 400ml unsweetened coconut milk
ice (optional)

1 Blend all the ingredients together and pour into a glass to serve. Top with a few extra fresh berries, if you have them, then drink up!

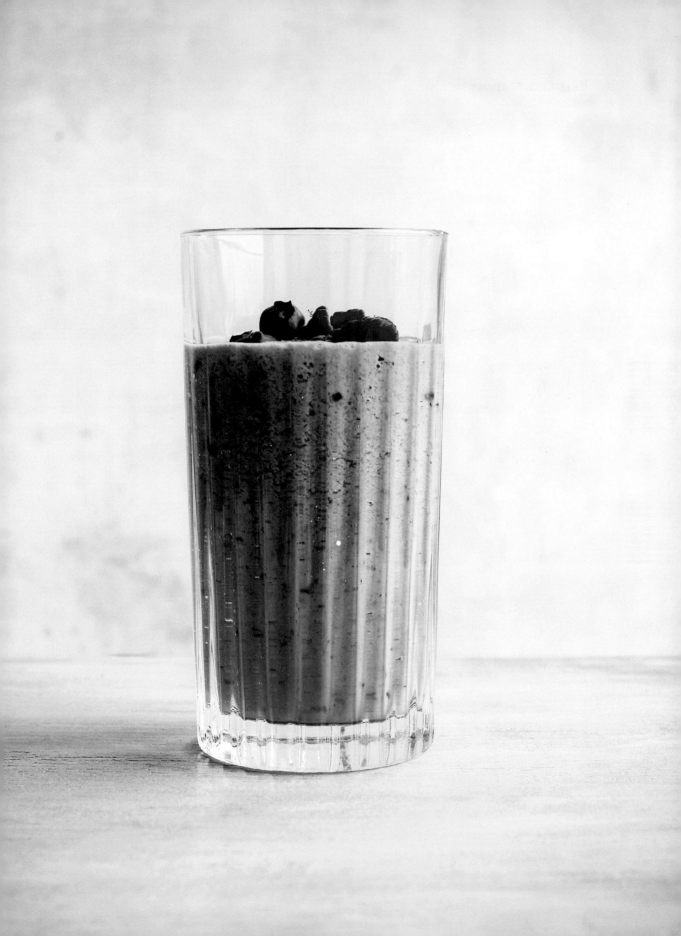

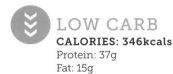

LOW CARB

CALORIES: 346kcals
Protein: 37g
Fat: 15g
Carbohydrate: 13g

Affogato Shake

I try to include a shake in every one of my plans as I know a lot of people have ZERO time in the morning. This one will definitely wake you up.

LOW CARB

1 scoop protein powder
    (chocolate, vanilla or coffee
    flavour would be best)
    (typically 25–30g)
170g 0% Greek yoghurt
    (typically 1 small pot)
    (Fage Total)
1 level tbsp cacao nibs
    (approx. 15g)
approx. 400ml unsweetened
    nut milk (any)
1 cup / shot strong, cold coffee
    (decaf, if preferred)
ice (optional)

1 Blend or shake all the ingredients together and drink up.

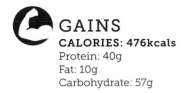

GAINS
CALORIES: 476kcals
Protein: 40g
Fat: 10g
Carbohydrate: 57g

Gains Shake

This shake is ideal to have pre- or post-workout.

GAINS
1 large handful / 1 sachet oats
   (typically 30g)
1 banana
1 scoop protein powder
   (typically 25–30g)
170g 0% Greek yoghurt
   (typically 1 small pot)
   (Fage Total)
approx. 400ml unsweetened
   nut milk (any)
ice (optional)

1 Blend all the ingredients together and drink up!

LOW CARB

CALORIES: 327cals
Protein: 37g
Fat: 12g
Carbohydrate: 15g

Chocolate Cake and Chocolate Sauce with Chocolate Sprinkles

This might seem a weird breakfast, but sometimes when I wake up, I just want something sweet! When cereal isn't an option, this can be a real saviour.

LOW CARB

1 scoop protein powder
(chocolate works best but any
will do) (typically 25–30g)
2 dashes unsweetened
coconut milk
170g 0% Greek yoghurt
(typically 1 small pot)
(Fage Total)
1 dash Sweet Freedom Choc Shot
(typically 5g)
1 tbsp cacao nibs (typically 15g)

1 Mix the protein powder and 1 dash of coconut milk together in a microwavable bowl to make a thick batter. Place the bowl in the microwave and cook on a high heat for 1½ minutes.

2 Meanwhile, mix the yoghurt, the second dash of coconut milk and the Choc Shot together in a small bowl.

3 Once the cake has cooked, pour the yoghurt sauce over the cake, sprinkle with the cacao nibs and serve.

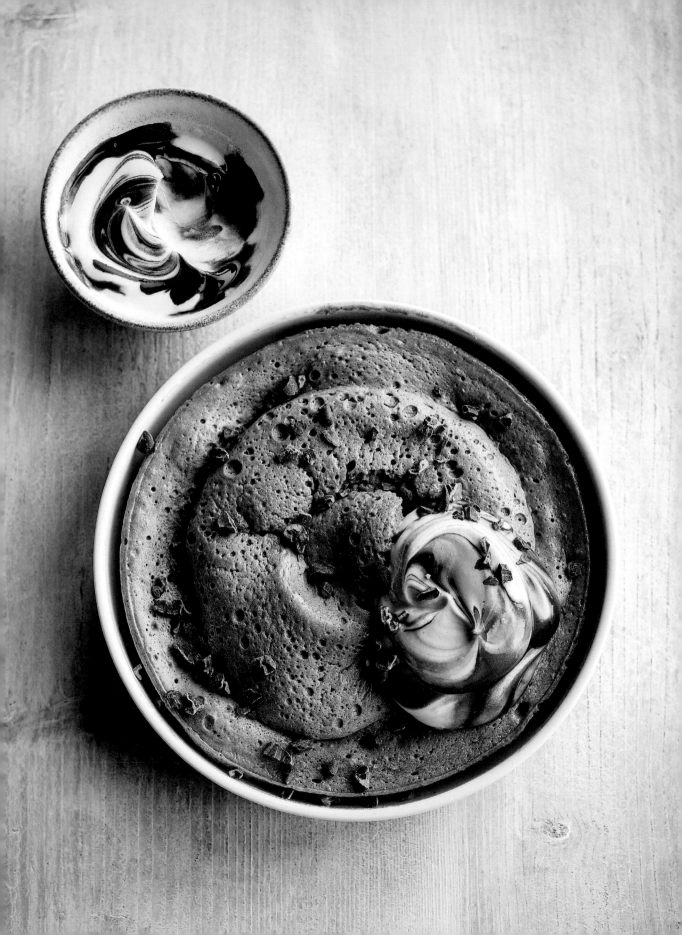

CALORIES: 303kcals
Protein: 22g
Fat: 17g
Carbohydrate: 13g

Nutella Bowl

Let's be honest, anything that combines hazelnut and chocolate is a winner, especially when you're on a diet!

LOW CARB

170g 0% Greek yoghurt (typically 1 small pot) (Fage Total)
1 tbsp crushed hazelnuts (approx. 15g)
1 tbsp cacao nibs (approx. 15g) (Myprotein)
1 swirl Sweet Freedom Choc Shot (approx. 5g)

1 Combine all the ingredients in a bowl and tuck in!

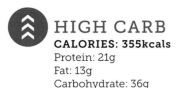

HIGH CARB
CALORIES: 355kcals
Protein: 21g
Fat: 13g
Carbohydrate: 36g

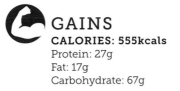

GAINS
CALORIES: 555kcals
Protein: 27g
Fat: 17g
Carbohydrate: 67g

Nutella Proats

Oats with Nutella? OK! I often have proats post-workout, hot or cold; they are an amazing hit of carbs and protein to help you refuel and recover.

HIGH CARB

1 large handful or 1 /sachet oats (typically 30g)
1 scoop protein powder (chocolate is best for this) (typically 25–30g)
2 level tbsp Nutella (approx. 30g)

GAINS

3 large handfuls or 3 sachets oats (typically 90g)
1 scoop protein powder (chocolate is best for this) (typically 25–30g)
2 level tbsp Nutella (approx. 30g)

1 Measure the oats and protein powder into a bowl.

2 Pour small amounts of boiled water into the bowl and stir as you go until you reach a consistency you are happy with. (I like my proats quite thick, but this is totally up to you.)

3 Stir half the Nutella into the oats, then dollop the remaining Nutella on top and serve.

CALORIES: 347kcals
Protein: 23g
Fat: 24g
Carbohydrate: 8g

Eggs Over Cheesy

I decided to lay these cheesy eggs on a bed of tomato and onion. Partly because cheese, tomato and onion go SO well together, but also because the added hit of fibre will be more filling and satiating.

 LOW CARB

2 whole eggs
40g Cheddar (approx. 2 slices)
1 tomato, diced
½ red onion, peeled and
    thinly sliced

1 Place a non-stick frying pan over a high heat and fry the eggs until the whites start to brown at the edges.

2 Flip the eggs, place the cheese on the cooked side and season with freshly ground black pepper. Leave the eggs to cook for a further 1–2 minutes.

3 Meanwhile, mix the tomato and red onion together in a bowl.

4 When the eggs are ready, remove them from the pan and place on top of the tomato and onion and serve wth a few rocket leaves, if you like.

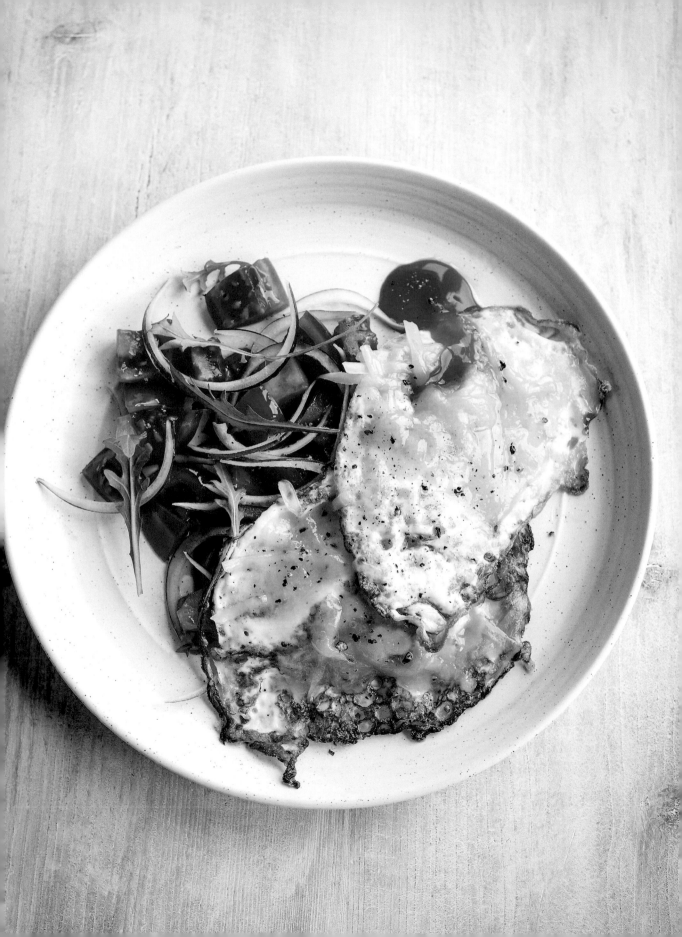

LOW CARB

CALORIES: 315kcals
Protein: 32g
Fat: 14g
Carbohydrate: 14g

Breakfast Stew

I like to come up with really filling, warming recipes that take the edge off dieting, and this is one of my all-time breakfast saviours!

LOW CARB

1 tsp olive (or chilli) oil
1 tsp diced or crushed garlic
½ onion, peeled and diced
2 chicken sausages (typically 34g each), sliced into discs (Heck Chicken Chipolatas)
½ × 400g tin chopped tomatoes
2 whole eggs
1 handful chopped fresh parsley, to serve

1 Place a frying pan over a high heat and add the oil.

2 When the oil is hot, stir in the garlic and onion.

3 Add in the sausage slices and toss everything together until all the ingredients are browned (typically 3–4 minutes).

4 Reduce the heat and stir in the chopped tomatoes. Bring to a simmer, then make 2 small dents in the stew with the back of a spoon. Crack the eggs into these dents and leave everything to cook gently for 10–15 minutes.

5 Spoon on to a plate, season with freshly ground black pepper, scatter with parsley and serve.

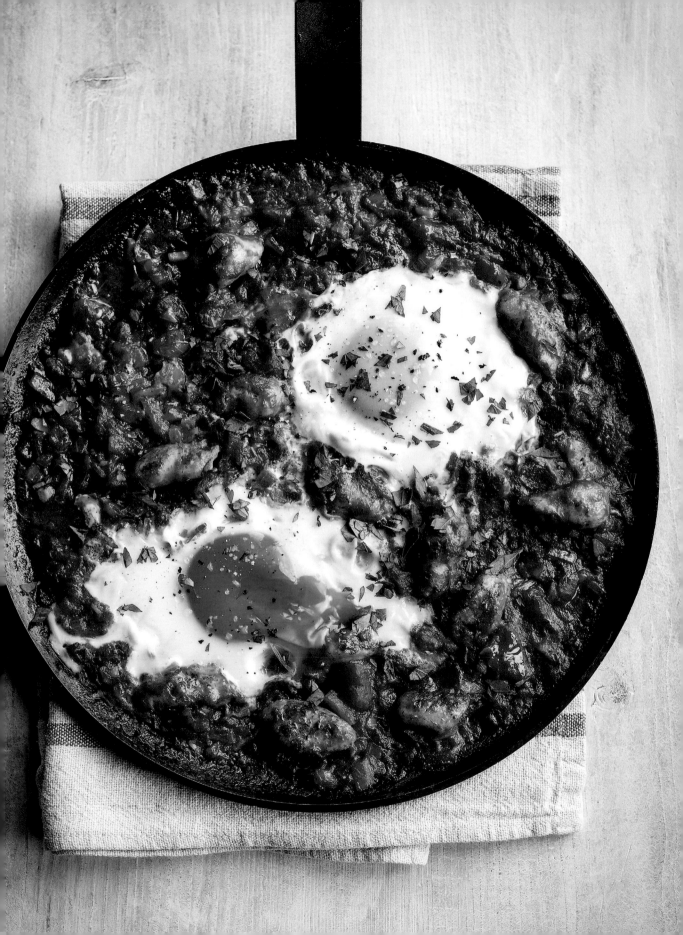

HIGH CARB
CALORIES: 349kcals
Protein: 22g
Fat: 12g
Carbohydrate: 33g

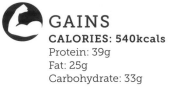 **GAINS**
CALORIES: 540kcals
Protein: 39g
Fat: 25g
Carbohydrate: 33g

Eggy Bread

This could be French toast, but I MUCH prefer it savoury, so eggy bread it is!
Adding bacon creates a higher calorie Gains version (pictured opposite)!
Season with black pepper and a pinch of paprika to serve.

 HIGH CARB

3 whole eggs
pinch of paprika (optional)
2 slices wholemeal bread (any)
2 tbsp reduced salt and sugar
    ketchup (Heinz)

GAINS

2 slices bacon (you can use any
    but I like smoked back bacon)
4 whole eggs
pinch of paprika (optional)
2 slices wholemeal bread (any)
2 tbsp reduced salt and sugar
    ketchup (Heinz)

1 If you're making a Gains stack of eggy bread, place a non-stick frying pan over a high heat and fry the bacon to the desired crispiness. Remove from the pan.

2 Crack the eggs into a bowl and whisk together well. Season with salt and pepper and paprika, if using. (You could use any other herbs and spices to flavour the egg.)

3 Place a slice of bread in the egg mixture and gently push down before turning it over and soaking the other side. Place a non-stick frying pan over a medium heat and cook the eggy bread for 2–3 minutes on each side (if you have already fried the bacon, use this pan). Repeat the process with the second slice of bread.

4 Remove from the pan, top with the bacon, if including, squirt with ketchup and serve.

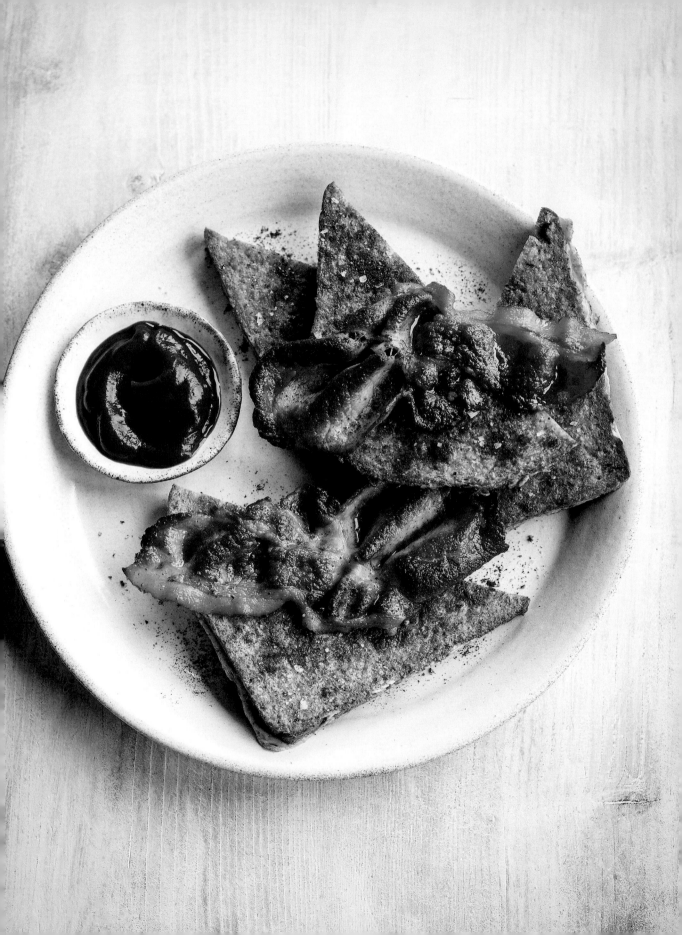

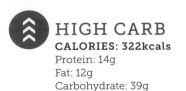 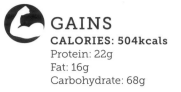

HIGH CARB
CALORIES: **322kcals**
Protein: 14g
Fat: 12g
Carbohydrate: 39g

GAINS
CALORIES: **504kcals**
Protein: 22g
Fat: 16g
Carbohydrate: 68g

Sweet Potato Hash

Filling, warming, and very, very healthy. I LOVE this recipe! Increase the sweet potato and egg quantities for a Gains Hash (pictured opposite).

HIGH CARB

1 tsp olive (or chilli) oil
1 tsp crushed or diced garlic
½ onion, peeled and diced
½ red pepper, diced
1 small sweet potato, chopped into small cubes (the smaller the better for quicker cooking time)
1 large handful spinach
2 whole eggs
pinch of chilli powder (optional)
pinch of paprika (optional)

GAINS

1 tsp olive (or chilli) oil
1 tsp crushed or diced garlic
½ onion, peeled and diced
½ red pepper, diced
2 small sweet potatoes, chopped into small cubes (the smaller the better for quicker cooking time)
1 large handful spinach
3 whole eggs
pinch of chilli powder (optional)
pinch of paprika (optional)

1 Pour the oil into a frying pan and place over a high heat.

2 When the oil is hot, add the garlic, then the onion and pepper and cook until softened (typically 3–4 minutes).

3 Add the sweet potato and toss all the ingredients together well. Reduce the heat slightly and cook until the potatoes are soft (typically 5–10 minutes), adding a splash of water if it's looking a little dry.

4 Add the spinach and cook until wilted.

5 Crack the eggs on to the top of the hash, cover the pan with a lid and allow to cook for a further 4–5 minutes.

6 Season with salt and pepper, then add the chilli powder and paprika, if using, and serve. (You could use any other herbs and spices to flavour your hash.)

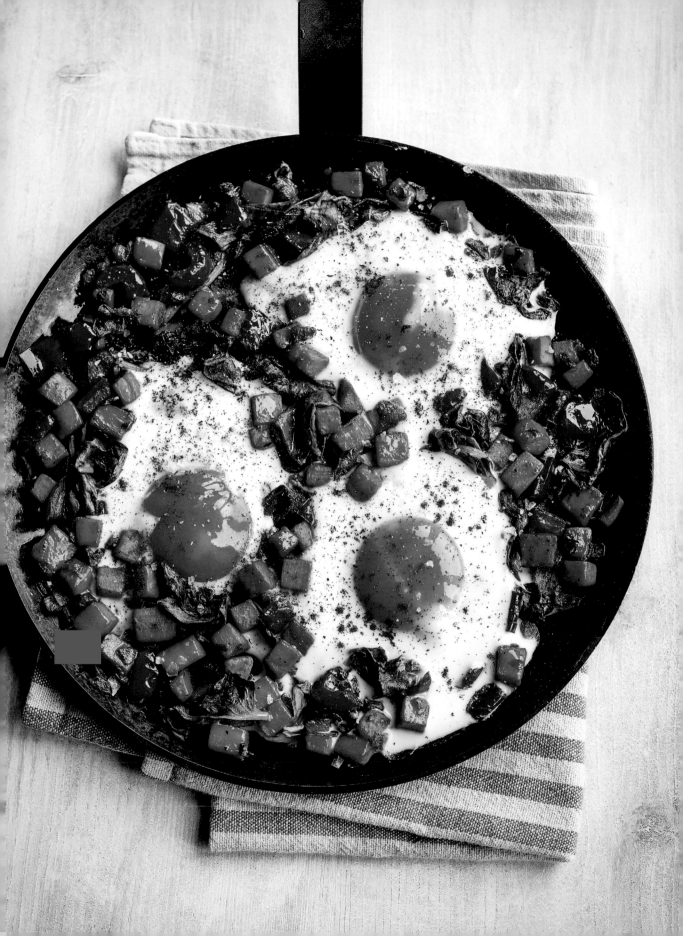

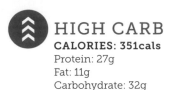 **HIGH CARB**
CALORIES: 351cals
Protein: 27g
Fat: 11g
Carbohydrate: 32g

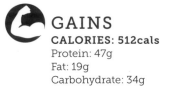 **GAINS**
CALORIES: 512cals
Protein: 47g
Fat: 19g
Carbohydrate: 34g

The Lean Sausage Butty

I'm from Manchester, so naturally the much fattier version of this was once a weekly staple! Add a couple of eggs for a great Gains Sausage Butty (pictured opposite).

HIGH CARB

1 tsp salted butter
2 chicken sausages (typically 34g each), cut lengthways to butterfly (Heck Chicken Chipolatas)
2 slices wholemeal bread (any)
1 squirt / 1 tsp reduced salt and sugar ketchup (Heinz)

GAINS

1 tsp salted butter
3 chicken sausages (typically 34g each), cut lengthways to butterfly (Heck Chicken Chipolatas)
2 whole eggs
2 slices wholemeal bread (any)
1 squirt / 1 tsp reduced salt and sugar ketchup (Heinz)

1 Melt the butter in a frying pan over a medium heat and place the butterflied sausages cut-side down in the pan. Leave to cook for 4–5 minutes then turn them over. If you're making a Gains Sausage Butty, crack the eggs into the pan and cook alongside the sausages for approximately 2–3 minutes. Remove from the pan with the sausages.

2 Place both slices of bread in the middle of the pan, allowing them to soak up the butter and sausage juices.

3 Turn up the heat to high and, when the bread starts to toast, remove from the pan and place on a plate.

4 Lay the sausages side by side on the bread, top with the egg, if including, squirt with ketchup, season with freshly ground black pepper and serve.

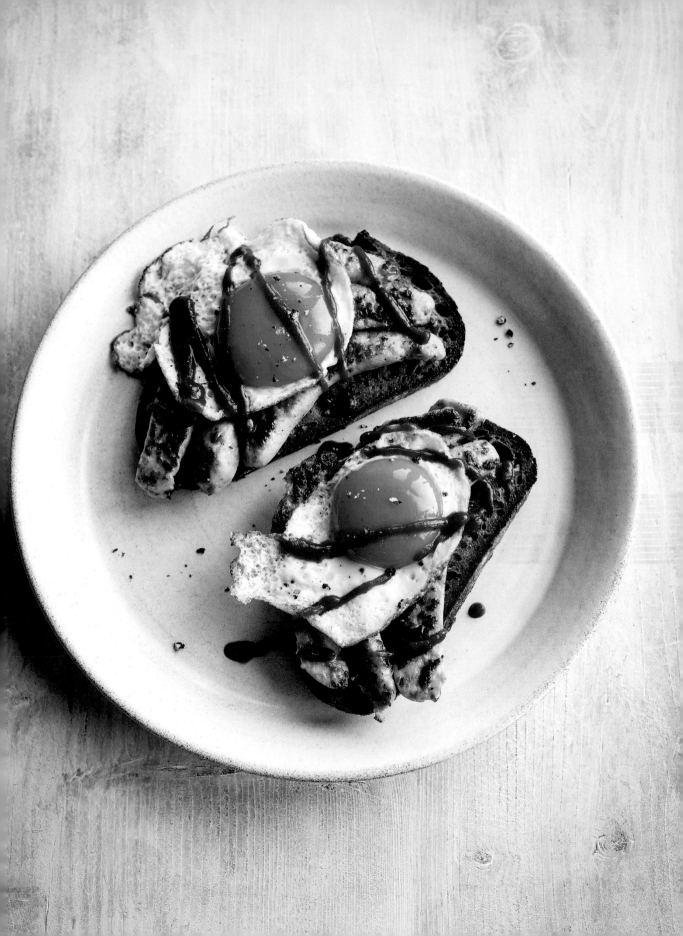

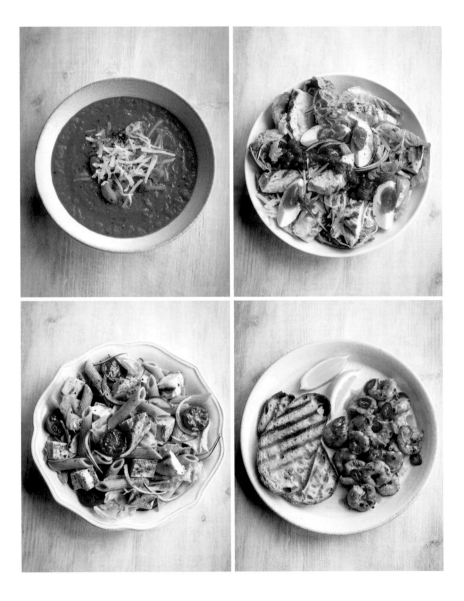

LUNCHES/ DINNERS

LOW CARB
CALORIES: 324kcals
Protein: 40g
Fat: 10g
Carbohydrate: 15g

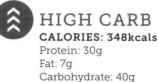 **HIGH CARB**
CALORIES: 348kcals
Protein: 30g
Fat: 7g
Carbohydrate: 40g

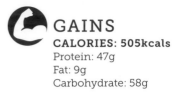 **GAINS**
CALORIES: 505kcals
Protein: 47g
Fat: 9g
Carbohydrate: 58g

Hearty Tomato Soup

My dad and I swear that it's tomato soup and NOT chicken soup for the soul! The low-carb version is pictured opposite – it's a truly comforting soup with a very subtle hit of protein. Adding some picked basil leaves would take it to another level!

LOW CARB

1 tsp olive oil
½ small onion, peeled and diced
1 small carrot, peeled and diced
1 small celery stick, diced
1 squirt / 1 tsp tomato purée
½ × 400g tin chopped tomatoes
400ml vegetable stock
100g Eat Lean Protein
   Cheese, grated

HIGH CARB

1 tsp olive oil
½ small onion, peeled and diced
1 small carrot, peeled and diced
1 small celery stick, diced
1 squirt / 1 tsp tomato purée
½ × 400g tin chopped tomatoes
400ml vegetable stock
60g wholewheat penne
   (dry weight)
60g Eat Lean Protein
   Cheese, grated

GAINS

1 tsp olive oil
½ small onion, peeled and diced
1 small carrot, peeled and diced
1 small celery stick, diced
1 squirt / 1 tsp tomato purée
½ × 400g tin chopped tomatoes
400ml vegetable stock
110g wholewheat penne
   (dry weight)
100g Eat Lean Protein
   Cheese, grated

1 Heat the oil in a large saucepan over a medium heat.

2 Add the onion, carrot and celery, season with salt and pepper and cook for 5–10 minutes until soft.

3 Reduce the heat to low, then stir in the tomato purée and tinned tomatoes.

4 Cover the pan with a lid and leave to simmer for 10–15 minutes.

5 Remove the lid to pour in the stock, then cover again and cook for a further 10–20 minutes, stirring occasionally.

6 If making a High-carb or Gains version, as the soup is cooking, boil the penne in a pan of salted water according to the packet instructions. Drain well.

7 Remove the pan of soup from the hob and, if you like, whizz with a hand blender until smooth.

8 Stir the cooked penne into the soup, if making a High-carb version.

9 Pour into a large bowl, sprinkle with the cheese and serve.

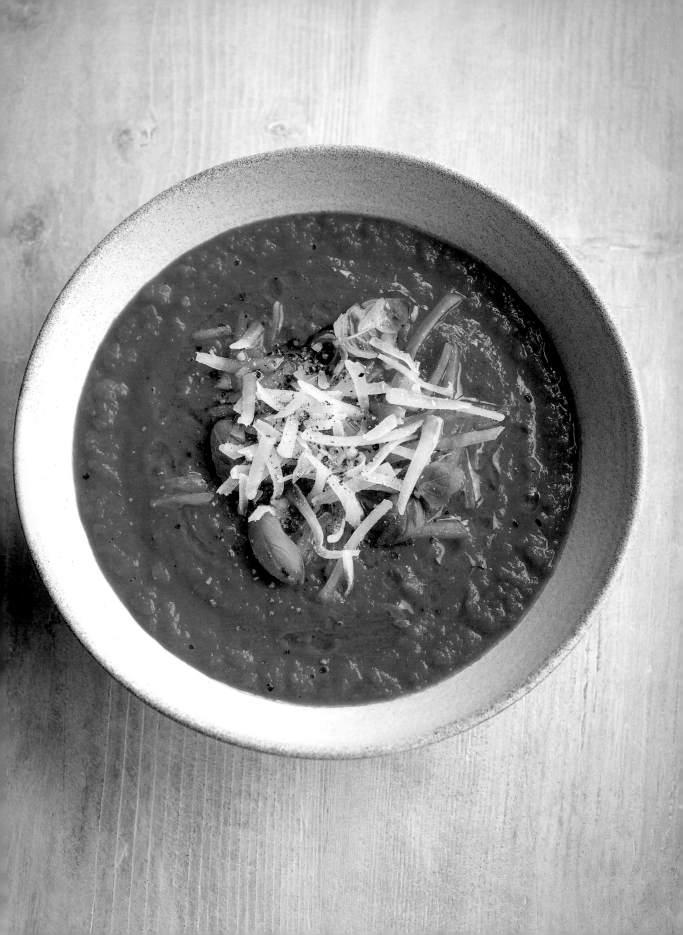

Is-This-Really-Healthy Salad

Salads aren't great unless they're full of warm, filling additions... Here is the best salad you will ever eat on a diet.

LOW CARB

1 chicken breast (approx. 125g)
1 whole egg
½ × 400g tin chopped tomatoes
1 Little Gem lettuce (any green salad leaf will do), leaves separated
½ red onion, peeled and diced or sliced
50g Eat Lean Protein Cheese, grated

1 Season the chicken breast and grill or fry in a non-stick pan until cooked through.

2 Meanwhile, boil the egg in a pan of water for 5–10 minutes, until slightly runny or hard-boiled, whichever your preference.

3 Place the tomatoes in another small saucepan, season with salt and pepper and simmer over a medium heat.

4 Place the lettuce in a large bowl with the onion and mix together well.

5 Remove the eggs from the pan, peel and slice into quarters. Cut the chicken into bite-sized pieces and add with the egg to the salad bowl.

6 Pour the hot tomatoes over the salad (I like to mix it in as a warm dressing).

7 Sprinkle the cheese over the top and serve.

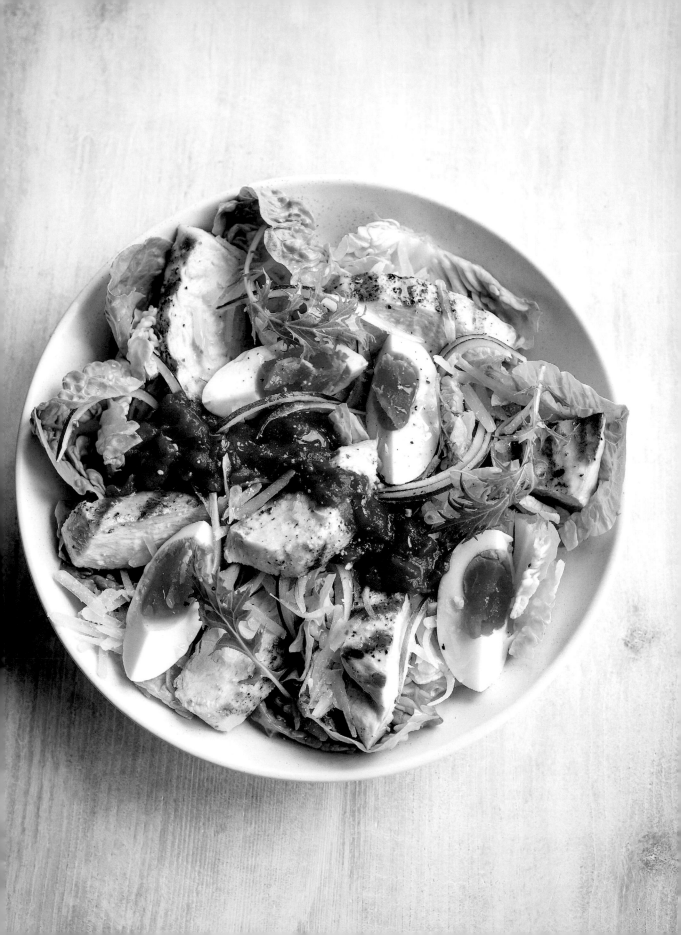

HIGH CARB
CALORIES: 316kcals
Protein: 29g
Fat: 8g
Carbohydrate: 30g

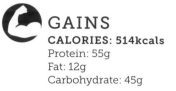 **GAINS**
CALORIES: 514kcals
Protein: 55g
Fat: 12g
Carbohydrate: 45g

Pasta Salad

This is my favourite high-carb salad to eat post-training!

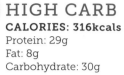 HIGH CARB

1 chicken breast (approx. 125g)
60g wholewheat penne (dry weight)
1 large portion iceberg lettuce (any green salad leaf will do), leaves torn
½ red onion, peeled and diced or sliced
5 cherry tomatoes, halved
1 tsp olive (or chilli) oil

GAINS

2 chicken breasts (approx. 125g each)
100g wholewheat penne (dry weight)
1 large portion iceberg lettuce (any green salad leaf will do), leaves torn
½ red onion, peeled and diced or sliced
5 cherry tomatoes, halved
1 tsp olive (or chilli) oil

1 Season the chicken breast(s) and grill or fry in a non-stick pan until cooked through.

2 Meanwhile, boil the pasta in salted water according to the packet instructions. Drain well.

3 Place the lettuce in a large bowl with the onion and tomatoes. Dice the cooked chicken and add to the salad bowl with the pasta.

4 Mix everything together well, season with salt and pepper, drizzle with the oil and serve.

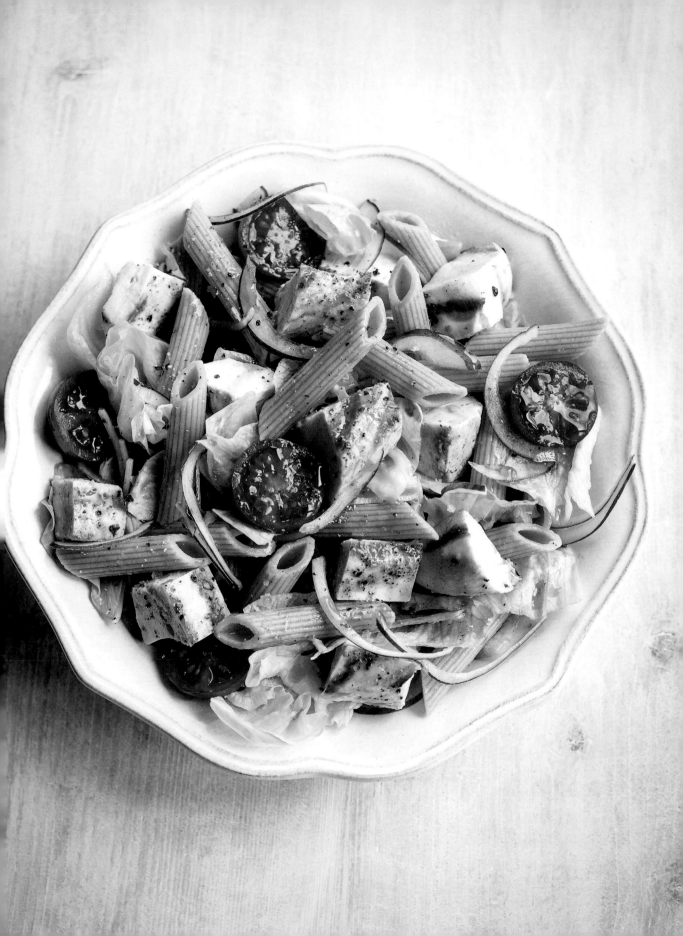

LOW CARB
CALORIES: 342kcals
Protein: 30g
Fat: 16g
Carbohydrate: 12g

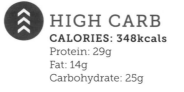 HIGH CARB
CALORIES: 348kcals
Protein: 29g
Fat: 14g
Carbohydrate: 25g

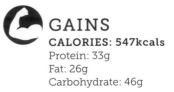 GAINS
CALORIES: 547kcals
Protein: 33g
Fat: 26g
Carbohydrate: 46g

Chicken Wrap

This is a warming wrap for when you're on the move. Lo-Dough is a GREAT tortilla alternative and is the perfect low-carb wrap – this recipe really hits the spot! Make two wraps using wholewheat tortillas for a great Gains meal (pictured opposite).

LOW CARB

1 chicken breast (approx. 125g), sliced into long, thin strips
1 piece Lo-Dough
2 level tbsp hummus (approx. 30g)
½ small cucumber, diced
1 small tomato, diced
½ small red onion, peeled and diced
1 tsp chilli oil
a few rocket leaves (optional)

HIGH CARB

1 chicken breast (approx. 125g), sliced into long, thin strips
1 wholewheat tortilla
1 level tbsp hummus (approx. 15g)
½ small cucumber, diced
1 small tomato, diced
½ small red onion, peeled and diced
1 tsp chilli oil
a few rocket leaves (optional)

GAINS

1 chicken breast (approx. 125g), sliced into long, thin strips
2 wholewheat tortillas
2 level tbsp hummus (approx. 30g)
½ small cucumber, diced
1 small tomato, diced
½ small red onion, peeled and diced
1 tsp chilli oil
a few rocket leaves (optional)

1 Season the chicken strips and fry in a non-stick pan over a medium heat for 6–8 minutes, tossing and turning occasionally, until cooked through.

2 Meanwhile, warm the Lo-Dough or wholewheat tortilla(s) in the microwave for 30 seconds. Remove from the microwave and spoon hummus into the centre and spread out evenly. Top with the chicken and diced veg then drizzle with chilli oil. Add the rocket, if using.

3 Fold the bottom of the wrap a little way over the contents, then roll into a tight wrap from right to left. Repeat with the other wrap, if you are making two.

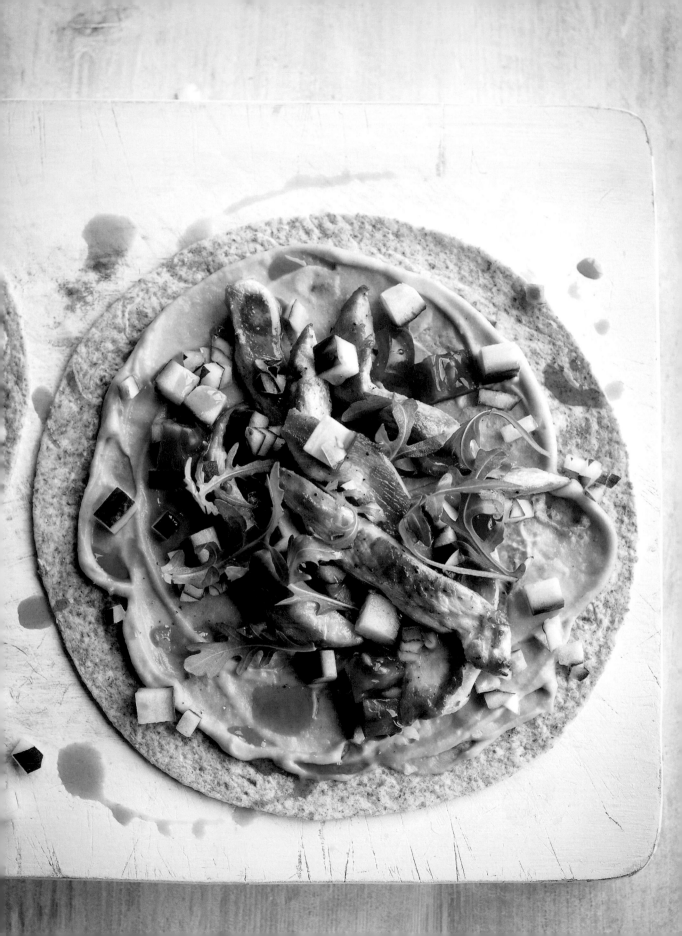

LOW CARB
CALORIES: 324kcals
Protein: 27g
Fat: 10g
Carbohydrate: 26g

HIGH CARB
CALORIES: 339kcals
Protein: 20g
Fat: 10g
Carbohydrate: 36g

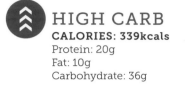

GAINS
CALORIES: 541kcals
Protein: 36g
Fat: 15g
Carbohydrate: 56g

Quorn Curry

Quorn is a great complete protein source and is not just for vegetarians – meat eaters can get a good hit of recovery with this recipe, too! Use 60g pilau rice (dry weight) for a High-carb meal and 120g pilau rice (dry weight) for a Gains meal. Scatter the finished dish with a handful of fresh coriander leaves and a few slices of green chilli, if you like your curry hot, and squeeze over some lime.

LOW CARB

1 tsp vegetable oil
150g Quorn pieces
½ onion, peeled and chopped
½ red pepper, deseeded and sliced
1 garlic clove, peeled and
    finely chopped
½ tsp ground ginger
1 tsp curry paste
½ × 400g tin chopped tomatoes
200g cauliflower rice

HIGH CARB

1 tsp vegetable oil
100g Quorn pieces
½ onion, peeled and chopped
½ red pepper, deseeded and sliced
1 garlic clove, peeled and
    finely chopped
½ tsp ground ginger
1 tsp curry paste
½ × 400g tin chopped tomatoes
60g pilau rice (dry weight)

GAINS

1 tsp vegetable oil
200g Quorn pieces
½ onion, peeled and chopped
½ red pepper, deseeded and sliced
1 garlic clove, peeled and finely
    chopped
½ tsp ground ginger
1 tsp curry paste
½ × 400g tin chopped tomatoes
120g pilau rice (dry weight)

1 Place the oil in a casserole dish over a high heat. Add the Quorn and cook for 5–10 minutes, depending on whether you are using fresh or frozen.

2 Add the onion, pepper, garlic and ginger and stir well. Leave to soften in the pan for 4–5 minutes.

3 Stir in the curry paste and pour in the tomatoes. Top with 100ml water and mix everything together well. Bring the curry to the boil, then reduce the heat and leave to simmer for 10–15 minutes, until the sauce has thickened to the desired consistency.

4 Meanwhile, cook the cauliflower rice (see below) or pilau rice according to the packet instructions.

5 Serve the curry on a large plate with cauliflower or pilau rice.

....

TIP: To make cauliflower rice, break a cauliflower into florets, place in a food processor and whizz, or grate with a cheese grater until riced. Season to taste. Warm in the microwave for 2–3 minutes on a high heat.

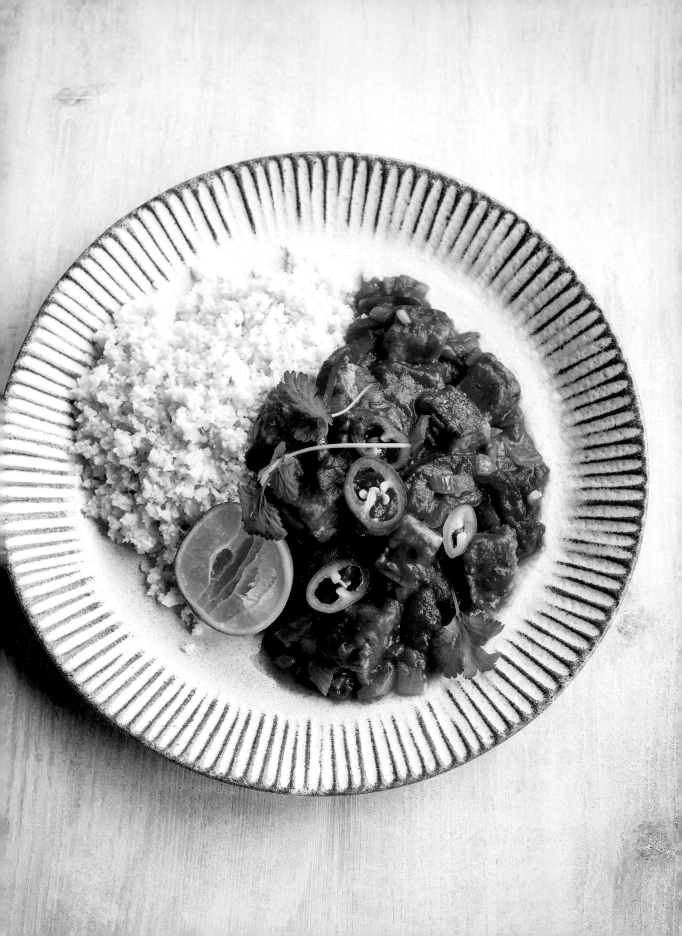

LOW CARB
CALORIES: 339cals
Protein: 20g
Fat: 27g
Carbohydrate: 2g

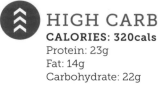 **HIGH CARB**
CALORIES: 320cals
Protein: 23g
Fat: 14g
Carbohydrate: 22g

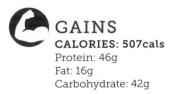 **GAINS**
CALORIES: 507cals
Protein: 46g
Fat: 16g
Carbohydrate: 42g

Prawns Pil Pil

My partner's all-time favourite snack and / or meal! The Gains version (pictured opposite) has been garnished with some sliced red chilli and is served with a couple wedges of lemon. Feel free to garnish the Low- and High-carb versions, too.

 LOW CARB

2 tbsp olive oil
2 garlic cloves, peeled and sliced
½ tsp chilli flakes
125g raw king prawns
juice ½ lemon

HIGH CARB

1 tbsp olive oil
2 garlic cloves, peeled and sliced
½ tsp chilli flakes
125g raw king prawns
juice ½ lemon
1 large slice crusty bread (any),
    griddled (optional)

GAINS

1 tbsp olive oil
2 garlic cloves, peeled and sliced
½ tsp chilli flakes
250g raw king prawns
juice ½ lemon
2 large slices crusty bread (any),
    griddled (optional)

1 Place the oil in a pan over a high heat and add the garlic and chilli flakes.

2 When the oil is spitting, add the prawns, season well with salt and pepper and toss continuously for 2–3 minutes until pink. (You could use any herbs and spices to flavour the prawns.)

3 Squeeze in the lemon and leave to simmer for another minute.

4 Pour the contents of the pan into a heated bowl and serve with griddled crusty bread, if using.

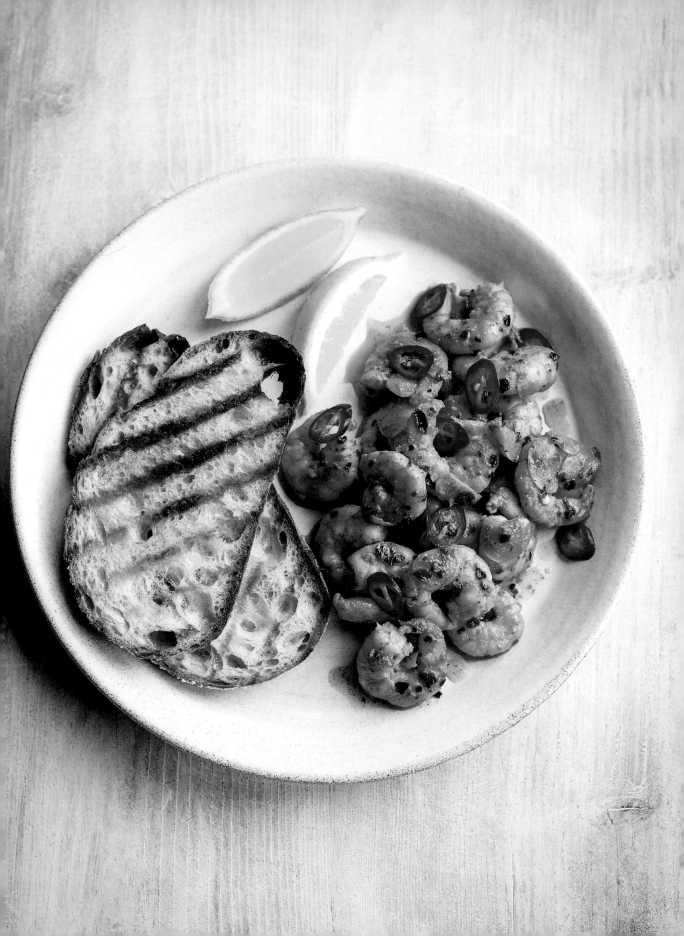

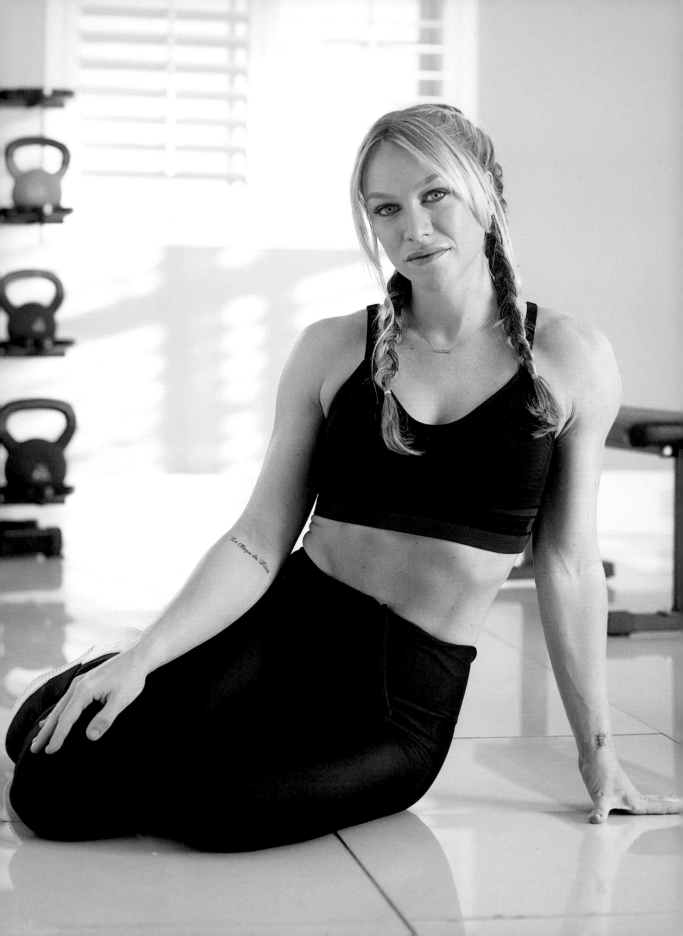

RECOVERY

This section will teach you how best to recover from your training, allowing both your lifting and aesthetic results to progress.

REST DAYS AND SLEEP

Rest days and sleep are just as important to physique results as training days.

While you *do* need to be in the gym lifting weights to see muscle growth – or on the treadmill doing cardio to see fat loss – you also need to allow your body to recover and rebuild.

As you will have seen in the weight-lifting plans, the training days cap at 6 times a week. Taking at least 1 **WHOLE** rest day a week is *imperative* for your results *and* your recovery.

However, I also encourage you to take rest days as and when you need them.

While DOMS (Delayed Onset Muscle Soreness) is part and parcel of a weight-lifting plan, *excessive* DOMS due to *excessive* training isn't optimal, and is a sign that you need a rest day (potentially 2 or 3 consecutively).

I recommend training anywhere between 4 and 6 times a week, and aiming to get as much sleep as possible each and every night.

Sleep routines are hugely important to both our internal and external health – I see both my training and my results suffer when my sleep patterns are all over the place. On a normal weeknight, I aim to be in bed by 10pm and up at 7am. When this pattern is disturbed, my sessions take a hit and the scales jump, and this is a *very* common theme among my clients.

Try to have a happy, healthy relationship with *both* your training *and* your recovery.

STRETCHING

It's pretty obvious that stretching is imperative both before and after training.

As I mention at the start of the stretching section on page 17, you should think of your body as a piece of chewing gum: if it's cold, it will snap in half; if it's warm, it's supple, and it will stretch.

If you go into a session cold and try to do a lift, *especially* a big compound lift like a squat, you are far more likely to get injured.

However, if you stretch dynamically (performing fluid movements and gentle bounces, for example) before you train, you will be warmed up, and not only will you be more likely to avoid injury, you will also find that you have a better range of motion in the lift itself.

Cooling down is just as important as warming up. As soon as you have finished your lift, repeat your warm-up stretching routine – only this time hold static poses.

A really good book to look into is ***Becoming a Supple Leopard*** by Glen Cordoza and Dr Kelly Starrett – many athletes swear by these techniques when it comes to both their performance and recovery.

If you:

» Train frequently

» Find that you often experience bad DOMS (Delayed Onset Muscle Soreness)

» Experience regular and / or severe stiffness

» Struggle with your range of motion in a lift

then you need to consider stretching as a much more *important* and *consistent* part of your daily routine.

Stretching needs to be something you really dedicate time to – from waking up in the morning, to other available times during your day, last thing at night and most *certainly* pre and post training. This may sound a bit of a nightmare, but I *promise* you will *feel* a million times better and you will *train* a million times better, too.

THERMOTHERAPY

Everybody knows that applying heat or cold to an injury or sensitive area can ease pain and reduce inflammation. However, the general, *lifestyle* application of thermotherapy by those who train and are looking to optimise their recovery is *greatly* underused.

When it comes to muscle or joint damage, basic heat therapy will *increase* blood flow to the injury site, helping it to relax and reducing pain. This improved circulation also helps your body eliminate any lactic acid waste left in the muscle after training, decreasing DOMS (Delayed Onset Muscle Soreness) and increasing recovery.

On the flip side, basic cold treatments reduce inflammation and pain by *decreasing* blood flow to the injured area. Rest, ice, compression and elevation (RICE) is a standard practice for injured athletes.

So how can you best increase your training and recovery using thermotherapy?

The Sauna

Not only has sauna use been proven to improve stress, anxiety and mood, it has also been proven to have *remarkable* effects on cardiovascular health as well as muscle growth *and* recovery.

The sauna has been proven to increase the hormone responsible for growth and recovery of every cell in the human body from two-fold to sixteen-fold, depending on the frequency of sauna use. It has also been extensively trialled and proven to increase longevity of life.

In short, if you want to improve your body's response to the stress of training, your overall mood, your cardiovascular health, your muscle growth and recovery, and your life...USE THE SAUNA.

Hot Water Immersion

Soaking in a hot tub or a hot bath (between 33–37.7°C / 92–100°F) will:

>> Warm up stiff muscles and tissues before physical activity

>> Decrease pain and discomfort of Delayed Onset Muscle Soreness (DOMS)

>> Encourage muscles to relax

>> Improve circulation and encourage your body to eliminate any lactic acid waste after training

Cold Water Immersion and Cryotherapy

I'm lumping these two together because, even though they are of course different methods, the intention of both is to prompt the exact same response in the human body... Cold Shock.

You are probably thinking *'Why the hell would I want to experience something called Cold Shock?'* but it has been proven to have some truly *astonishing* effects on the human body...

>> Improved focus and mood (via increased norepinephrine hormone)

>> Increased fat burning (via increased mitochondria in adipose tissue)

>> Improved physical performance in training (via increased mitochondria in muscle tissue)

Whether you induce this state by taking ice baths or by spending time in a Cryo Chamber, the effects can greatly improve both your **response to** and **recovery from** training.

A FINAL WORD

I hope that you find weight lifting to be as fun and rewarding as I have found it to be.

A few things to remember:

» Always focus on form first. Only turn your focus to progression – added weight and / or volume (sets and reps) – once your form is right.

» Switching up your lifting goals (endurance, hypertrophy and strength) and variation in exercises are going to improve your results and progress.

» Recovery is just as important as training. Days off, good sleep, good nutrition, hydration, stretching, supplementation and appropriate recovery techniques will all greatly help you to progress as the weeks, months and years pass.

As long as you take care of your body, the sky is the limit in the gym.

INDEX

ACKNOWLEDGEMENTS

Thank you to my literary agent, Clare Hulton, who knew I wanted to write a weight-lifting book from day one and never took her eyes off the prize!

Thank you to Transworld for letting me write this book, in particular my favourite dream-team-trio; Michelle Signore, Emma Burton and Becky Short.

Thank you to Jo Roberts-Miller and Emma and Alex Smith for making this book come to life – you guys are insanely talented!

Thank you to Meera and Sam for putting up with me on shoot days and getting me through each and every exercise with a smile on my face and a flapjack in my hand!

Thank you to my husband, James Haskell. All three of my books have marked a significant period in our relationship, from weddings to retirements and overseas adventures. I am thrilled that I get to do this life stuff with you by my side.

Thank you to my small group of best friends who have watched this all unfold from side lines and cheered me on (even though none of you care about fitness or nutrition and you're eagerly awaiting my dietary retirement!).

Thank you to my family – my mum, dad, three brothers, three sisters-in-law, two nieces and one nephew. You guys are my home, my heart, and my perspective. Thank you for letting me hold your children, even when we all know I might break them.

And, as always, the best are saved for last … Thank you to my amazing Blitzers, followers and Bodcast listeners for your constant interest, support and excitement. I value each and every one of you, and I thank you from the bottom of my heart for allowing me to do what I love.

★ ★ ★

All the equipment I used in the photos is by PULSE FITNESS. If you are interested in purchasing any fitness equipment whatsoever (from a mat, to a dumbbell, or even a Smith machine) for your home or gym, Pulse can provide, deliver and set up your desired space. You can find them at: **http://thepulsegroup.co.uk/pulse-fitness**.